Childbirth - Clinical Assessment, Methods, and Management

Edited by Panagiotis Tsikouras, Nikolaos Nikolettos, Werner Rath and Friedrich Von Tempelhoff

Published in London, United Kingdom

Childbirth - Clinical Assessment, Methods, and Management
http://dx.doi.org/10.5772/intechopen.111304
Edited by Panagiotis Tsikouras, Nikolaos Nikolettos, Werner Rath and Friedrich Von Tempelhoff

Contributors
Adriana Elena Ghelmene, Aise Chatzi Ismail Mouchterem, Alexios Alexiou, Anastasia Bothou, Dimitrios Kyriakou, Dusica Lecic-Tosevski, Efthimios Oikonomou, Georgios Iatrakis, Guillermo Valenzuela, Konstantinos Nikolettos, Kristina Roloff, Maja Milosavljevic, Manuela Cristina Russu, Natalia Sahnova, Nektaria Kritsotaki, Nikolaos Nikolettos, Panagiotis Tsikouras, Ruxandra Viorica Stănculescu, Snezana Rakic, Sonia Kotanidou, Stefani Filiou, Suryani Manurung, Theopi Nalbanti, Tijana Vranes, Tina Bui, Triada Charmanidou, Vlassis Spanakis, Xanthoula Anthoulaki, Yoko Kato, Şerban Nastasia

First published in London, United Kingdom, 2024 by IntechOpen
IntechOpen is the global imprint of INTECHOPEN LIMITED, registered in England and Wales, registration number: 11086078, 5 Princes Gate Court, London, SW7 2QJ, United Kingdom
Printed in Croatia

British Library Cataloguing-in-Publication Data
A catalogue record for this book is available from the British Library

Additional hard and PDF copies can be obtained from orders@intechopen.com

Childbirth - Clinical Assessment, Methods, and Management
Edited by Panagiotis Tsikouras, Nikolaos Nikolettos, Werner Rath and Friedrich Von Tempelhoff
p. cm.

This title is part of the Obstetrics and Gynecology Book Series, Volume 1
Topic: Maternal-fetal Medicine
Series Editor: Zouhair O. Amarin
Topic Editor: Artúr Beke

Print ISBN 978-0-85014-174-0
Online ISBN 978-0-85014-175-7
eBook (PDF) ISBN 978-0-85014-176-4
ISSN 3049-706X

For EU product safety concerns:
IN TECH d.o.o., Prolaz Marije Krucifikse Kozulić 3, 51000 Rijeka, Croatia,
info@intechopen.com or visit our website at intechopen.com.

IntechOpen Book Series

Obstetrics and Gynecology

Volume 1

Aims and Scope of the Series

Obstetrics and Gynecology field typically covers several subspecialties that include maternal-fetal medicine, gynecologic oncology, reproductive endocrinology and subfertility, urogynecology and female pelvic reconstructive surgery, critical care medicine, complex family planning, pediatric and adolescent gynecology, menopausal and geriatric gynecology, and minimally invasive gynecologic surgery.
Apart from being diverse, obstetrics and gynecology is a challenging and demanding specialty. It combines medical and surgical skills.
The sequence of books in this series will have certain characteristics in common that will be recognized as part of the same informative multi-volume book programme.

Meet the Series Editor

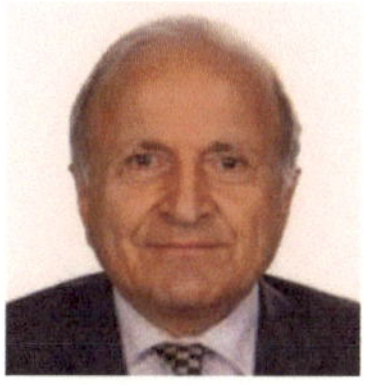

Zouhair Amarin is a Professor of Obstetrics and Gynaecology at the Jordan University of Science and Technology. He was previously a lecturer at the University of Glasgow, Scotland, a senior lecturer at the University of Nottingham, England, and the dean of the Faculty of Medicine at Mutah University, Jordan. Professor Amarin is a fellow of the Royal College of Obstetricians and Gynaecologists, and the Faculty of Public Health, London. He holds master's degrees in medical science and medical education. He is a pioneer in IVF and was the first in the world to develop microsurgical epididymis sperm aspiration for clinical use. He also discovered a surgical procedure for critical ovarian hyperstimulation syndrome. Professor Amarin has edited books, authored book chapters, and published more than 130 papers. He is the recipient of eight awards.

Meet the Volume Editors

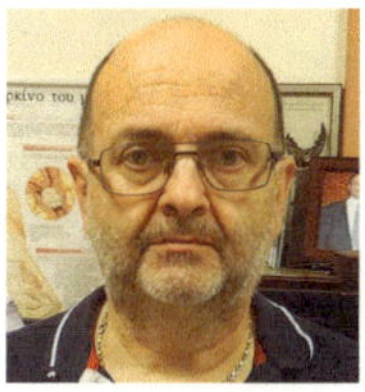

Panagiotis Tsikouras is a specialist in obstetrics and gynecology, perinatal medicine, and contraception at the School of Medicine, Democritus University of Thrace, Greece. He is also head of the Family Planning Centre and Gynecological Cytology Laboratory at the same university. Dr. Tsikouras is a fellow of the International Academy of Clinical and Applied Thrombosis/Hemostasis. His scientific activities focus on pediatric and adolescent medicine, gynecological oncology, and high-risk pregnancies. He is a reviewer for several international journals and has numerous scientific publications to his credit, including papers and book chapters. He has also contributed to international and national guidelines on coagulation and thrombosis in obstetrics and gynecology.

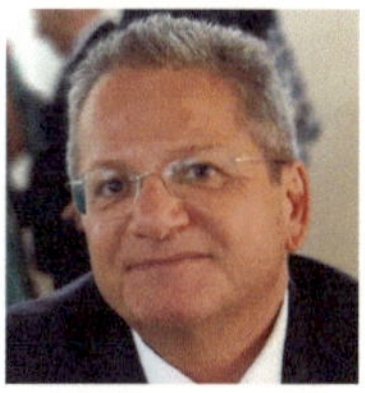

Prof. Nikolaos Nikolettos is a Professor of Obstetrics and Gynecology and Assisted Reproduction at the Democritus University of Thrace, Greece. He has training in gynecological endocrinology, human reproduction, and in vitro fertilization. From 2007 to 2011, he was the director of the In Vitro Fertilization Unit, University Regional General Hospital of Alexandroupolis, Greece. From 2012 to 2018, he was the director of the Laboratory of Reproductive Physiology-Artificial Fertilization. In 2019, he took over the management of the University Obstetrics-Gynecology Clinic of the Medical Department at the Democritus University of Thrace. His scientific work includes more than 100 publications in international journals and numerous invited lectures at international and Greek conferences.

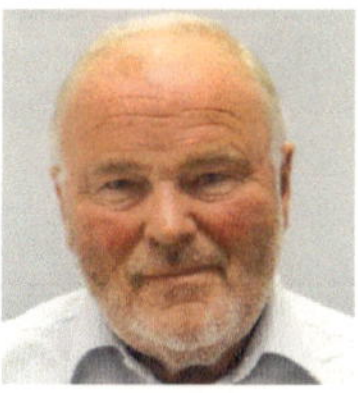

Prof. Dr. h. c. Werner Rath is a specialist in obstetrics and gynecology, gynecologic oncology, perinatal medicine, and hemostaseology. He was chief of the Department of Gynecology and Obstetrics, University Hospital Aachen, Germany. He is a Professor of Gynecology and Obstetrics in the Faculty of Medicine, University Kiel, Germany. He received an honorary doctorate from the University of Alexandroupolis, Greece. Dr. Rath is the recipient of several awards, including the Staude-Pfannenstiel Award of the North Germany Society of Gynecology and Obstetrics, Maternité Award from the German Society of Perinatal Medicine, and the Berlin Harald-Bräutigam Award. He is a reviewer for numerous journals.

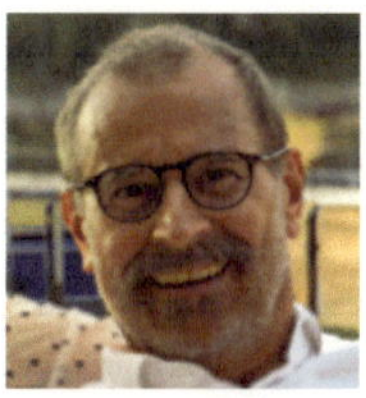

Prof. Dr. Freidrich von Tempelhoff, FCATH, is a specialist in obstetrics and gynecology, gynecologic oncology, perinatal medicine, and hemostaseology. He is chief of the Department of Gynecology and Obstetrics and head of the Institute for Thrombosis and Coagulation Disorders in Gynecology and Obstetrics, Teaching Hospital Vinzencius Hospital, Hanau Germany. He completed his medical education at Justus-Liebig University, Germany, and became a Consultant of Obstetrics and Gynecology in 1996. In 1993, he received his doctorate in medicine and completed his habilitation at the Johannes-Gutenberg University Mainz, Germany in 2007. He was appointed extracurricular professor at the Julius-Maximilians-Universität Würzburg, Germany in 2015. He is a fellow of the International Academy of Clinical and Applied Thrombosis/Hemostasis. His scientific focus is on hemostaseological and hemorheological disorders in women with miscarriages, preeclampsia, and thrombosis. Dr. Tempelhoff is a reviewer for numerous journals, author of several publications and book chapters, and a contributor to international and national guidelines on coagulation and thrombosis in gynecology.

Contents

Preface

Spontaneous childbirth is a phenomenon that leads to the exit of the fetus, placenta, and membranes from the pelvic cavity of the pregnant woman through the vagina. Childbirth is achieved with the necessary condition of periodic, involuntary, painful contractions of the uterus. A necessary condition for understanding childbirth is the knowledge of three factors: the uterus, the pelvic canal, and the fetus. The duration of pregnancy is genetically predetermined while it is also influenced by the environment.

The fetus is born after the end of its normal maturation, however, the factors that cause labor to occur in a full-term pregnancy have not been fully elucidated. Placental corticotropin acts in the fetoplacental unit, which creates a suitable endocrine environment for the initiation of labor through the pituitary–adrenal axis and the placenta.

In the mother, changes in the function of the placenta due to the increased concentration of pro-inflammatory factors (cytokines and interleukins) create the appropriate hormonal environment, while the synthesis of prostaglandins and oxytocin facilitates the response of the myometrium and cervix.

During pregnancy, contractions of the myometrium take place with the action of estrogens and prostaglandins, but initially, they do not spread throughout the body of the uterus. Later in pregnancy, intercellular connections between the smooth muscle fibers in the myometrium are progressively established, and as the electrical activity is transmitted from cell to cell, the myometrium contracts in a coordinated and localized manner, and Braxton Hicks contractions occur.

At the onset of labor, oxytocin circulates in high concentrations in the mother and its receptors develop on the surface of the smooth muscle cells of the uterus. Prostaglandins enhance the action of oxytocin, while estrogens facilitate the production of prostaglandins from the placenta. Other factors such as interleukin and cytokines further facilitate the coordinated activity of the myometrium at the onset and duration of labor.

Some cases of labor not progressing may be due to a lack of synchronization between cervical ripening and myometrial contractions.

Although many of the factors involved in the initiation of labor affect both the myometrium and cervix in different ways, oxytocin is a hormone that acts almost exclusively on the myometrium and has little effect on the cervix.

The diagnosis of labor is of great importance, as the incorrect diagnosis can lead to iatrogenic interventions that may not be needed or even to complications. For the diagnosis of labor, there must be the start of regular uterine contractions and progressive changes in the cervix.

However, the diagnosis of regular uterine contractions (labor pains) is quite problematic, as is their differential diagnosis from Braxton Hicks contractions. That is why the diagnosis of labor is made by examining the cervix and the upcoming changes in it. Friedman's graphic representation that laid the foundation for modern labor monitoring practice uses changes in the cervix to define the latent and active phases of the first stage of labor.

Contractions are manifested by the appearance of periodic contractions of the uterus and are intended to dilate the cervix, exit the fetus, and detach and exit the placenta and membranes. Each contraction shows a beginning, a peak, and a decline.

The intensity of the contraction is assessed clinically by placing the palm on the abdomen of the patient. The resting stage of the uterus also varies. The contraction frequency is the number of contractions within a certain time interval. The expected normal range is three to five contractions every 10 minutes. Along with the clinical assessment, continuous recording of the contractions is done with the help of an electronic head, which is placed on the abdomen of the pregnant woman (external tocography) or, more rarely, by placing an intra-amniotic catheter (internal tocography). The contractions and the birth must be treated in the way chosen by the obstetrician in consultation with the midwife. There are many decisions to be made, so the obstetrician must be aware of every possible option.

The contribution of attending physicians and midwives is important in dealing with problems that may arise during labor and birth. Access to information and practical and moral support are equally important. If both parents attend the relevant childbirth classes, they will be better informed and actively more supportive. This book is a manual with useful information for those practicing obstetrics in the "trenches" who need real advice on how to deal with real problems. It is a modern, practical reference guide to help solve problems of everyday obstetric practice.

Panagiotis Tsikouras
Professor,
Department of Obstetrics and Gynecology,
Democritus University of Thrace,
Alexandroupolis, Greece

Nikolaos Nikolettos
Professor,
Department of Obstetrics and Gynecology,
Democritus University of Thrace,
Alexandroupolis, Greece

Werner Rath
Professor,
Gynecology and Obstetrics in the Faculty of Medicine,
University of Kiel,
Kiel, Germany

Friedrich Von Tempelhoff
Professor,
Gynecology and Obstetrics,
St. Vinzenz Teaching Hospital,
Hanau, Germany

Section 1

Prenatal Assessement of Pregnancy

Chapter 1

Cervical Length and Perinatal Outcome

Panagiotis Tsikouras, Triada Charmanidou, Stefani Filiou, Georgios Iatrakis, Anastasia Bothou, Efthimios Oikonomou, Dimitrios Kyriakou, Aise Chatzi Ismail Mouchterem, Alexios Alexiou, Konstantinos Nikolettos, Nektaria Kritsotaki, Theopi Nalbanti and Nikolaos Nikolettos

Abstract

Prematurity nowadays has taken on significant dimensions. It is a complex medical issue with socio-economic consequences. The estimation of cervical length, assessed during the second trimester of pregnancy, using transvaginal ultrasound, may help to reduce rates of prematurity. By predicting the risk of preterm birth and identifying women who are at high risk of preterm birth, certain practices could be implemented, such as the use of progesterone or cerclage placement. Nonetheless, it remains unsolved the question of certain strategies, such as the use of progesterone in pregnant women with shortened cervical lengths. This work examines the relationship of cervical length during pregnancy to the perinatal outcome.

Keywords: cervical length, cervical cerclage, Arabin pessary, perinatal outcome, cervical funneling, medical treatment

1. Introduction

Prematurity is defined as labor before the completion of 37 weeks of gestation is globally a major factor in infants' morbidity and mortality. It has been estimated that annually almost 15 million premature infants are born, consisting of about 11% of all the laborers globally. 85% of these cases are infants that have completed 32–36 weeks of gestation, 10% are infants that have completed 28–31 weeks of gestation and 5% are infants that are extremely premature which means the ones who do not have completed 28 weeks of gestation [1–4]. Prematurity seems not only to result in 1.000.000 deaths annually but also to be the leading cause of infants' death. The percentage of morbidity related to prematurity is also high, as huge as the number of financial resources that must be spent in this public health sector [1–4].

The most important risk factor of prematurity is the existence of an obstetric history of prematurity. Nonetheless, the prediction of premature birth is not an easy task due to its complexity. Various well-known risk factors for preterm birth in singleton pregnancies have emerged from many studies. Among other risk factors of prematurity are also multiple pregnancies [1–4].

What is more, the ultrasonographic estimation of cervical length before 24 weeks of gestation in singleton pregnancies is implemented during the second trimester of pregnancy. Studies show the inverse relationship between cervical length and preterm delivery, and since cervical length ultrasound assessment is a safe, reliable, and repeatable method, its use has been established in the second trimester of pregnancy aiming the detection of pregnancies at increased risk for premature birth and to the implementation of secondary prevention practices, which will be discussed later in this text. It has been estimated that women in triplet pregnancy with a cervical length < 25 mm between 15 and 24 weeks of gestation have a 51% risk of preterm delivery before the 32nd week of gestation. While in women that are at low risk of preterm birth and with the estimated risk of preterm birth in this population to be 4% (singleton pregnancies, absence of history of preterm birth in previous pregnancy), a correlation appears to exist between preterm birth and cervical length, measured by ultrasound between 19th and 24th week of pregnancy. In these singleton low-risk pregnancies it has been found that a cervical length of 15 mm occupies the third percentile, having a sensitivity of 8.2% and a specificity of 99.7% in the prediction of preterm birth below 32 weeks of gestation, with a cervical length of 25 mm corresponding to the tenth percentile in pregnancies of 16–24 weeks of gestation (threshold below which the cervix is described as "short") [5–10].

Furthermore, the risk of preterm birth appears to be higher when the detection of short cervical length occurs earlier in pregnancy. In addition, it is particularly interesting that the presence of a short cervix may somehow be added to other risk factors for preterm birth. For example, the combination of obstetric history of preterm birth and short cervix has a relative risk for preterm birth of 3.3, higher than the one that appears in pregnancies in which there is only a short cervix. Thus, it has been suggested by various organizations, such as ACOG, for women with a history of preterm birth to have their cervical length measured from the 16th to 24th week of pregnancy, while the question of whether it is worth applying the same practice to low-risk women is still controversial. The latter view is based on various studies suggesting that only a small proportion of low-risk, based on obstetric history, pregnant women will be able to be identified by ultrasound assessment of their cervical length (from the 5% of the primiparous women that eventually will give birth prematurely, only 23.3% of them have a short cervix in mid-pregnancy ultrasound). Another study found that although women with a cervix <25 mm give birth prematurely more frequently than women with cervical length > 25 mm calculated at mid-pregnancy, the vast majority of women with premature labor (82%) do not show a short cervix in the second trimester of pregnancy. Given the association between this cervical length in the second trimester of pregnancy and the risk of preterm birth, various medical practices have been proposed and studied, which are also applied in everyday clinical practice to prevent premature birth. The use of progesterone, cervical pessaries, and cervical cerclage each individually or all in combination used to treat "short" cervix, especially in singleton pregnancies, has raised many questions about the usefulness of these practices as measures to treat premature birth and also about the effectiveness of the above-mentioned treatment options [10–15].

Progesterone, the most researched and well-known technique of preterm birth prevention, can be administered in singleton pregnancies with a history of preterm delivery between 16 and 36 weeks of gestation at a dosage of 250 mg once weekly (17-OHPC), 200–400 mg orally, or 100–200 mg vaginally daily [10–15]. Studies have shown that administering progesterone via intravaginal or intramuscular injections of 17-hydroxyprogesterone from the second trimester of pregnancy through the third significantly lowers the risk of preterm birth in women with "short" cervixes, whether or not they have a prior history of preterm birth. However, as far as high-risk women are concerned, there are studies, such as OPPTIMUM (multicenter, double-blind randomized study) that based on their data there is no statistically significant reduction in the risk of preterm delivery with intravaginal progesterone administration. Therefore, more evidence is expected in this field to demonstrate the benefit of progesterone to each group of women and the most effective route of its administration [10–15].

The aim of this study was to collect information on the deduction of results concerning the relationship between cervical length and perinatal outcome. Although cervical length during the second trimester of pregnancy can be a helpful tool for identifying women who have a high risk of preterm birth, the current study concentrated on the cervical length, estimated by ultrasound between 20 and 22 weeks of gestation, and the risk of preterm birth in singleton pregnancies. Moreover, the present study was not only limited to singleton low or high-risk pregnancies for preterm birth but also included data concerning the relationship between cervical length and risk of preterm birth in twin and triplet pregnancies.

What is more, this study tried to examine the importance of cervical length measurement in the first trimester of pregnancy in the estimation of preterm birth risk. Such a relationship could be really useful since this would allow earlier medical intervention for the prevention of preterm birth.

Also, this study presented the relationship between cervical length in the third trimester of pregnancy and perinatal outcome (time of spontaneous onset of labor, success rates of labor induction). Those all are matters that highly concern obstetricians nowadays [10–15].

Generally, the aim of this study was through the review of the literature, the recognition of the women who are at high risk for preterm birth, and the implementation of strategies that could eventually prevent preterm birth.

2. Method

The search was made through Medline, Pubmed, EMBASE, and Cochrane Library using as keywords the following expressions: transvaginal ultrasound in pregnancy, transvaginal evaluation of cervix during pregnancy, mid-trimester evaluation of the cervical length, cervical length and prematurity, cervical assessment in twin pregnancy, cervical evaluation in triplet pregnancies, cervical length in the first trimester of pregnancy. The studies that were used in the present study examined the relationship between cervical length in the first, second, and third trimesters of singleton, twin, and triplet pregnancies and the risk of preterm birth.

The next step was to categorize all the relative studies that were gathered, based on some common characteristics of each subgroup study population. So, the following subcategories of studies were created: cervical length during the second trimester of singleton pregnancies and risk of prematurity. Cervical length during the first trimester-early second trimester of pregnancy and correlation with mid-trimester cervical length and risk of prematurity. Cervical length during the third trimester of pregnancy and prediction of spontaneous onset of labor, prediction of the risk of caesarian section, and success rates of labor induction. All the studies that were related to one of these subcategories were examined further.

3. Results and discussion

Preterm birth, or the delivery of infants before 37 weeks of gestation, is a major contributor to neonatal morbidity and mortality and is therefore a problem with socioeconomic implications. It has been estimated that about 41,000 premature babies are born every day worldwide. Morbidity and mortality rates resulting from preterm birth are higher for "early" preterm infants (<28 weeks) and moderate preterm infants (28–32 weeks) and lower for "late" preterm infants (33–36 weeks). Since prematurity is associated with the appearance of various short- and long-term complications in neonates, such as retinopathy, cerebral hemorrhage, necrotizing enterocolitis, respiratory distress syndrome, neurodevelopmental disorders, one can easily understand the dimensions of this medical topic of prematurity [16–20].

Mortality rates appear to reach 44% for neonates 23 weeks old, 32% for 24 weeks old neonates, 12% for 25 weeks old neonates, 11% for 26 weeks old neonates, 8% for 27 weeks old neonates, and 2% for 28 weeks old neonates. The causes of death in preterm infants can be sometimes not clear and in each case, it is unclear which specific factor ultimately led to premature death. Often, neonates that end up in intensive care units for premature neonates have no other recognized cause of death than that of the general title of preterm delivery [16–20].

In Canada, these percentages have been translated into real costs and money that have to be spent in this sector of health. Specifically, the two-year survival rate was found to be 56% for "early" preterm infants, 92.8% for "moderate" preterm infants, and 98.4% for "late" preterm infants. Also, the mean hospitalization time for moderately preterm infants varied from 1.6 days at the age of 2 years to 0.09 days at the age of 10 years. The cost per neonate for the first 10 years of their life resulting from the above data is estimated to be $ 67,467 for an "early" preterm neonate, $ 52,769 for a moderate preterm neonate, and $ 10,010 for a "late" preterm neonate. So, the national amounts, if we take into consideration the above costs, would be $ 123.3 million for "early" preterm infants, $ 255.6 million for moderately preterm infants, $ 208.2 million for "late" preterm neonates, and $ 587.1 million for all the newborns. So, based on the above medical and financial data, the importance of finding and adopting early prevention programs is fully understandable [16–20].

This can theoretically be achieved through the application of programs of cervical length measurement in the second trimester of pregnancy and its association with the risk of preterm labor. Such programs aim to identify and characterize women as high risk, in which "short" cervical length in combination with other characteristics from women's obstetric history will lead to the subsequent implementation of practices that will prevent preterm birth, leading to a significant reduction in prematurity rates.

Transvaginal ultrasound examinations of the cervical length have been shown to accurately predict preterm labor in both asymptomatic low-risk women and those who are already showing signs of preterm labor. Also, several studies have examined the use of transvaginal ultrasonography in high-risk asymptomatic women with significant differences to be noted between these studies regarding the cervical length that is considered as pathological, pregnancy age at which the measurement should be performed, and the gestational age that preterm labor eventually happens.

Several meta-analyses have examined the association between transvaginally measured cervical length and the prediction of preterm birth in asymptomatic women with singleton or multiple pregnancies. A systematic review of Crane, which included a sample of 2258 high-risk asymptomatic women with singleton pregnancies, concluded that there was an inverse relationship between cervical length and the possibility of preterm labor. The cervical threshold under which the cervix was considered to be short was set at 25 mm, predicting with high sensitivity the risk of premature birth below 35 weeks of gestation, while women with a prior history of preterm labor and cervical surgery were identified as high risk for preterm labor. It was also found that the likelihood of preterm birth below 35 weeks is less in cases where cervical length < 25 mm is measured at 20–24 weeks of gestation, than the likelihood of preterm labor in cases where cervical length < 25 mm is measured at a gestational age less than 20 weeks or more than 24 weeks [20–24].

The women with a history of automatic onset of preterm birth included in the above analysis did not differ from those women who were getting into premature labor after premature rupture of fetal membranes and automatic onset of rhythmic contractions. And since the pathogenetic mechanisms in these two broad categories of preterm birth differ significantly, the predictive value of transvaginally measured cervical length was examined separately in these two subgroups. Some of the studies used in this analysis included a variety of risk factors for preterm birth, such as maternal age and smoking. These risk factors did not appear to have the same predictive value as other risk factors, such as history of previous preterm birth and presence of abnormalities in the uterus, so a subsequent statistical analysis was performed in this study and found that the results of the analysis were still the same even after exclusion of Watson's study that included smoking in older women in risk factors [24–28].

Previous studies have also noted the association between cervical surgeries and preterm labor. In Crane's meta-analysis, however, it was found that in women with a history of cervical surgery, cervical length less than 25 mm measured below 24 weeks of gestation was predictive of preterm birth before 35 weeks of gestation. Cervical length measured by transvaginal ultrasound at 24 weeks of gestation was found to be correlated with preterm labor before 37 weeks of gestation, but not with preterm labor before 34 weeks of gestation. In addition, this study showed that a cervical length less than 25 mm may be used as a predictive tool for preterm birth in women who have undergone correction surgery for uterine abnormalities. Last but not least, it was found that the most frequently used gestational age for cervical length ultrasound assessment and prediction of preterm birth is 20–24 weeks [28–32].

In a systematic review study, which included a sample of 1593 women and aimed to assess the accuracy of transvaginally measured cervical length during the second trimester of pregnancy in the prediction of preterm birth in twin pregnancies, it was found that this method of transvaginally measured cervical length works as a better predictor of preterm birth in twin pregnancies than in singleton pregnancies. For this reason, based on the analysis of Honest, women with singleton pregnancies and cervical length at 22–24 weeks of gestation less than or equal to 25 mm exhibited sensitivity and specificity in predicting preterm delivery below 32 and 34 weeks of pregnancy 4.2 and 0.4 and 4.4 and 0.67, respectively, while asymptomatic women with twin pregnancies and cervical length at 20–24 weeks of gestation below 20 mm exhibited sensitivity and specificity in predicting preterm delivery below 32 and 34 weeks of gestation 10.1 and 0.64 and 9.0 and 0.64, respectively [28–32].

Although the present study has, among other things, highlighted the value of transvaginally measured cervical length in the prediction of preterm birth in twin pregnancies, the efficacy of therapeutical practices that are based on the results of such studies and that are aiming to prevent premature birth is not certain. It is critical to note at this point that there is currently no therapeutic method that effectively seems to prevent premature birth in twin pregnancies, as it has been suggested in singleton pregnancies the implementation of practices such as cervical cerclage and progesterone.

4. Cervical cerclage

Cervical cerclage is effective in reducing the risk of preterm birth in high-risk pregnancies. Studies have proven that it contributes to statistically significantly fewer premature births before 33 weeks of gestation.

Specifically, in women with cervical cerclage, the rate of deliveries before 33 weeks was 13% compared to 32% observed in women without cervical cerclage Furthermore, a meta-analysis of randomized trials investigating the effectiveness of ultrasound-guided cervical suture placement in women with a history of second-trimester miscarriage or preterm delivery concluded that deliveries before 35 weeks' gestation were statistically significantly less in cases where suture cervical cerclage was placed compared to cases where some other treatment was followed (RR 0.57; 95% CI 0.33, 0.99 and RR 0.61; 95% CI 0.40, 0.92, respectively). Thus, cervical suture placement as a means of preventing preterm delivery in singleton pregnancies is indicated according to the guidelines in the following cases [32–36]:

History of one or more second-trimester miscarriages associated usually in a future pregnancy with painless cervical dilation and absence of signs of labor or rupture of fetal membranes. History of cervical cerclage in a previous pregnancy due to painless dilatation of the cervix during the second trimester. Painless cervical dilatation was found on physical examination. Ultrasound findings in combination with a history of preterm delivery, i.e. preterm delivery before 34 weeks in a previous pregnancy and cervical length in the current pregnancy below 25 mm as found in an ultrasound check before 24 weeks of pregnancy [36–40].

However, the effectiveness of placing a suture around the cervix of women carrying twins is not entirely certain also, whether the indications for cervical suture placement in twin pregnancies are equivalent to those in singleton pregnancies is still under investigation.

A study comparing selective cervical ligation with simple observation, but without determining whether and what risk factors were present, found no statistically significant difference between the two comparison groups. This result is similar to that of singleton pregnancies where routine cervical cerclage in all pregnancies without appropriate case selection has been found to offer no benefit [36–40].

A meta-analysis of randomized trials involving the use of cervical suture ligation in both singleton and twin pregnancies according to cervical length and setting a threshold of less than 15 mm in singleton pregnancies and less than 25 mm in twin pregnancies concluded that in singleton pregnancies with a positive history, there was a statistically significant benefit in reducing the risk of delivery before 35 weeks (RR 0.74, 95% CI 0.57, 0.96). When there was a miscarriage or premature birth in the second trimester in the history, the probability of risk was even lower (RR 0.57 and 0.61, respectively). However, in twin pregnancies without a positive history, it was seen that cervical ligation increased by 2 times the risk of delivery before 35 weeks of gestation (RR 2.15, 95% CI 1.15, 4.01). This result, however, comes from a single study that included a small number of cases, although it is reasonable to conclude that the placement of a cervical cerclage suture in twin pregnancies in which a short cervical length is found in a random check without the presence of a history, does not offer a benefit. However, the possible benefit of twin pregnancies with a short cervical length and the presence of risk factors has not yet been clarified.

Furthermore, placing a cervical ligation suture in women with twin pregnancies due to a cervical length of less than 25 mm before 24 weeks gestation and using the sequential cervical length measurement approach found that ligation may clinically significantly reduce preterm birth before 34 weeks compared with conservative management such as bed rest (36.7% in the band group vs. 50% in the rest group) [36–42].

This study demonstrated that suture ligation in twin pregnancies does not harm but instead provides a benefit when cervical length decreases on consecutive ultrasound measurements. Data on the placement of suture cervical cerclage in twin pregnancies with a history of preterm birth or second-trimester miscarriage are unfortunately lacking.

5. Cervical cerclage suture placement techniques

Cervical cerclage is defined as the placement of a suture in the cervix to maintain the pregnancy, which can be done through a transvaginal or transabdominal surgical approach. The two transvaginal techniques for ligation are the modified McDonald and the Shirodkar but without finding superiority of one over the other technique. Also, no superiority of one type of non-absorbable suture over another has been found, so the type of suture is freely chosen by the clinician. In the McDonald surgical technique, a simple non-absorbable suture is placed circularly in the cervix at the level of the cervical junction. Retrospective studies have found no benefit in placing a second suture to reinforce or reconstruct the cervical mucosa.

The Shirodkar technique involves the preparation and detachment of the cervical mucosa from the cyst in order to place the suture as close as possible to the height of the internal cervical os. To achieve this, the bladder and rectum are prepared and detached from the cervix, a non-absorbable suture is placed as close as possible to the internal cervical os, and the knot is then covered with mucosa [36–42].

Transabdominal suture placement at the level of the cervical isthmus is preferred in women in whom there is an indication for suture placement but the transvaginal approach is not possible due to anatomical problems (such as after cervical ectomy) or failure of transvaginal suture placement Transabdominal suture placement can be performed either open or laparoscopically depending on the surgeon's clinical experience.

Usually transabdominal banding is done at the end of the first trimester or at the beginning of the second trimester (between 10 weeks and 14 weeks of pregnancy) or before pregnancy and can remain between pregnancies in cases where the delivery is completed by cesarean section [36–42].

6. Administration of progesterone: intramuscular administration of progesterone

Intramuscular administration of 17-alpha hydroxyprogesterone is considered to be effective in preventing preterm delivery in singleton pregnancies with a positive history of preterm delivery. Regarding twin pregnancies, intramuscular administration of 17-alpha hydroxyprogesterone 500 mg twice weekly can approximately four-fold reduction in delivery before 32 weeks gestation (RR 3.78, p < 0.001) but cannot reduce the risk of delivery before 37 weeks gestation (RR 1.06, 95% CI 0.75, 1.51) [36–42].

However, no benefit was seen in neonatal-perinatal outcomes when intramuscular progesterone was compared with sham treatment. Thus, at present intramuscular progesterone is not recommended in twin pregnancies, although it would be of particular interest to further clarify its administration in a high-risk group pregnant.

7. Vaginal administration of progesterone

Vaginal progesterone appears to reduce the risk of preterm delivery. In a statistical meta-analysis of randomized trials that administered vaginal progesterone to asymptomatic pregnant women with shortened cervical length, vaginal progesterone was found to reduce delivery before 28 weeks of gestation (RR 0.51; 95% CI 0.31, 0.85), before 33 weeks of gestation (RR 0.56; 95% CI 0.31, 0.85) and before 35 weeks of gestation (RR 0.67; 95% CI 0.51, 0.89) [36–42].

Also, the use of vaginal progesterone was associated with a reduction in neonatal mortality and morbidity (RR 0.59; 95% CI 0.38, 0.91). Despite the fact that this tendency was not statistically significant, preterm birth at 33 weeks of gestation was found to be less likely in asymptomatic women with a cervical length of less than 25 mm in the second trimester of pregnancy. Also, the use of vaginal progesterone is associated with a 48% reduction in neonatal mortality as well as in the incidence of neonatal complications (RR 0.52; 95% CI 0.29, 0.93). In twin pregnancies, however, vaginal progesterone has been found not to reduce neonatal mortality and mortality (RR 0.97; 95% CI 0.77, 1.2). It is important to note, however, that in selected cases and with a cervical length below 25 mm before 24 weeks of gestation, vaginal progesterone can significantly reduce neonatal mortality and the incidence of neonatal complications (RR 0.56; 95% CI 0.42, 0.75) [42–46].

The daily recommended dose of progesterone is 90 mg in gel form and 200 mg in vaginal tablets (100 mg twice daily). The efficacy of higher doses of progesterone (400 mg) in reducing preterm birth and neonatal mortality and morbidity has not been proven. There appears to be a trend, but not statistically significant, of an increased incidence of cholestasis of pregnancy in a subgroup of women who received higher doses of progesterone.

8. Vaginal pessary

Placement of a ring-shaped plastic around the cervix vaginally has been used to prevent preterm birth for over 50 years, with greater interest being gained since 2003, when it was found that after placement of the pessary in pregnancies there were no preterm births. Thirty-two weeks gestation in a follow-up study of high-risk pregnancies for preterm delivery where a vaginal pessary was placed, delivery before 37 weeks was observed in 50% of women. However, in a randomized study that included singleton pregnancies with a cervical length of 25 mm or less, the rate of preterm delivery in pregnancies who had a pessary inserted was 6%, compared to 27% observed in pregnant women where only follow-up was performed (OR 0.18, 95% CI 0.08, 0.37) [42–46].

In twin pregnancies with a cervical length below the 25th percentile, vaginal pessary use reduced both preterm delivery (before 32 weeks' gestation) and poor perinatal outcome. Specifically, prematurity was 14% in the vaginal pessary group versus 29% in the monitoring group (RR 0.49, 95% CI 0.24, 0.97), while poor perinatal outcome was 2% in the vaginal pessary group versus 29% in the monitoring group (RR 0.4, 95% CI 0.19, 0.83). The results were even more encouraging in the subanalysis of high-risk pregnancies for the occurrence of preterm birth [42–50].

9. Combination of therapeutic approaches

In a systematic review and statistical meta-analysis that included both randomized and non-randomized studies, it was found that only seven studies could be included in the review, which only involved singleton pregnancies, and there was no data on twin pregnancies.

This review found that there was no difference in reducing the risk of preterm delivery before 34 weeks gestation when the combination therapy including vaginal pessary and progesterone was compared with pessary monotherapy (RR 1.3, 95% CI 0.7, 2.42) or administration of progesterone (RR 1.16, 95% CI 0.79, 1.72). In addition, there was no difference in the reduction of preterm birth before 37 weeks gestation when the combined treatment of cervical banding and progesterone administration was compared with cervical banding alone (RR 1.04, 95% CI 0.56, 1.93) or progesterone administration. (RR 0.82, 95% CI 0.57, 1.19) [48, 51–54].

However, as mentioned above, these data are limited and related to singleton pregnancies, while there is no data on twin pregnancies.

Since the 22nd week of gestation and every 2 weeks, there was a steady gradual decrease in the cervical length of the study population. The pattern of this decrease was even present in women who did not eventually give birth before 32 weeks of gestation, and this finding was consistent with existing literature data [48, 51–54]. Ramin observed that this decline became apparent after the 20th week of pregnancy, while Hiersch observed a faster rate of cervical length reduction in triplet pregnancies compared to that noted in twin pregnancies. However, a sharp decrease in cervical length from the 22nd to the 24th week of gestation appeared to be specific to triplet pregnancies that are at increased risk for preterm delivery between 24 and 32 weeks of gestation.

Although in many studies in triplet pregnancies, a short cervix is characterized the one that is less than 25 mm, with a cervical length of 34–35 mm, with sensitivity and specificity of 60–80% and 70–90% respectively, considered as critical in this study. A study conducted by Mheen is one of the few in which the cervical length limit has been set to 30 mm. By applying this limit, however, a predictive accuracy of 87.4% has been achieved. Ideally, this accuracy would reach 100%, something previously attempted through the acceptance of the 20 mm threshold between 25 and 28 weeks of gestation, a limit, though, inconsistent with the findings of the current study. Wherever the "critically short" cervical threshold is set in the various studies, it is advisable to keep in mind that women with shorter cervical lengths may have already been led to miscarriages in the second trimester of pregnancy or to preterm birth and therefore not being included in the sample of the study population. However, all described cervical length limits appear to be relevant in clinical practice, and none of them should be considered more accurate and significant than others [48, 51–54].

Concerning the chorionity of the triplet pregnancies, no significant difference was found in cervical lengths. Thus, chorionity was excluded from the prognostic parameters for preterm birth below 32 weeks of gestation in this study, which is not in the AMPHIA study, and the study of Perdigao and colleagues. Therefore, as far as the chorionicity in multiple pregnancies is concerned, it is important to deduct more studies with larger numbers of samples to draw safer conclusions [48, 51–54].

The usefulness of measuring the cervical length at different stages of pregnancy has been investigated in addition to doing so during the second trimester of pregnancy using transvaginal ultrasonography. There is a relatively small number of studies evaluating the sensitivity of the cervical length measured before the 16th week of pregnancy in predicting preterm birth, with the results being controversial [54–58].

Studies by Naim, Berghella, and Andrews found a strong association between short cervical length and preterm labor. A study by Hassan found that a "short" cervix at 14–19 weeks is a weaker predictor of preterm birth than an ultrasound assessment of cervical length in mid-pregnancy. Contradictory results were presented by Hasegawa, as well as by Zorzoli, who found in their studies no association between "early" cervical ultrasound assessment and preterm birth [54–58].

Conoscenti in a study with a sample of 2469 women with singleton pregnancies measured cervical length at 13–15 weeks of pregnancy aiming to calculate the risk of preterm birth. It was found that the average gestational age at birth was 40 weeks, with the incidence of preterm birth being 1.7%. In this study, early risk factors, such as previous history of preterm birth, were found to be consistent with those of other studies, and the main finding of this study was the inability to predict women who would eventually be led to premature birth since cervical length was similar to women who gave birth at term compared to the ones who gave birth prematurely, regardless of the presence of risk factors. In other words, the cervical length measured at 14 weeks of gestation appeared in this study, similar between women at high risk of preterm birth and women at low risk [54–58].

This finding is also not in accordance with other studies that show a strong relationship between cervical length's shortening in mid-pregnancy and a history of previous second-trimester miscarriages or preterm births. A possible explanation for this may be the association of a history of previous preterm birth with the risk of preterm birth, a finding presented also by Heath, who recorded apparent cervical lengthening alterations, after mid-pregnancy in the second trimester of pregnancy. A study conducted by Greco, with a sample of 9974 singleton pregnancies and with ultrasonographic cervical length assessment at 11–13 weeks of gestation to assess the risk of preterm birth, found that labor before 34 weeks of gestation, concerning 1% of the study population, could be predicted at 54.8% (95% CI 44.7–64.6) and with false negative rates of 10%, by combining cervical length with various features of the pregnant woman.

A similar study conducted by Sananes, with a sample of 31,834 pregnancies, seemed to detect at 23.3%, with a 10% false negative rate, preterm birth, which accounted for 3.7% of the study population, by ultrasound assessment of cervical length in the first trimester of pregnancy. In another study by Carvalho, cervical length was estimated in the first (11–14 weeks) and second trimester (22–24 weeks) of pregnancy in a random population of singleton pregnancies. The mean cervical length at 11–14 weeks of gestation was found to be 42.4 mm and 38.6 mm at 22–24 weeks of gestation. These findings of the above-mentioned study are consistent with those of other studies. In a study by Zalar, an ultrasound assessment of cervical length in the first trimester of pregnancy (11.3 ± 1.9 weeks) revealed an average cervical length of 46 mm in a low-risk population of pregnant women. In another study by Kushnir, which included 166 low-risk preterm labor women, cervical length was measured at 8–13 weeks of gestation and found to be 43 mm. Moreover, in a study by Guzman, cervical length assessment was performed in 469 high-risk preterm labor women with continuous ultrasound measurements between 14 and 24 weeks of gestation. Thus, the cervical length was found to be shorter at 21–24 weeks of gestation than at 15–20 weeks of gestation [54–58].

Cervical length during the first trimester of pregnancy, as shown by the above studies, appears to be even longer than that of non-pregnant premenopausal women. This could probably be explained by understanding the role that the lower part of the uterus plays in the cervical segment in the first trimester of pregnancy.

Carvalho observed that cervical length showed a gradual shortening from the first to the second trimester of pregnancy. This decrease in cervical length, however, was more obvious in the group of women who eventually had preterm birth. Cervical length ranged from 42.7 to 39.3 mm in women who gave birth at term, whereas in women who gave birth prematurely, cervical length decreased from 40.6 mm at 11–14 weeks of gestation to 26.7 mm at 22–24 weeks of pregnancy. Given these data, in the group of the women that will have premature birth, the decrease in cervical length occurs between the first and second trimester of pregnancy, and the degree of cervical shortening is related to the degree of prematurity. Guzman has also described this model of cervical shortening, presenting the weekly rate of cervical shortening between 15 and 24 weeks of gestation in women at high risk of preterm birth. To establish the ultrasonographic diagnosis of cervical insufficiency it was necessary in this study to find a progressive decrease in cervical length below 20 mm before 24 weeks gestation. Sufficient cervices showed a non-significant decrease in cervical length (−0.3 mm/week) compared to "insufficient" cervices (−4.1 mm/week, $P < 0.001$). In a study presented by Murakawa, which evaluated the cervical length in 32 women with threatened preterm labor and in 177 normal singleton pregnancies between 18 and 37 weeks of gestation, it was found that cervical length in women with threatened preterm labor was even shorter in women who also had history of preterm birth (23.2 mm compared to 31.7 mm in women with a free history of prematurity) [58–62]. In addition to looking at the significance of cervical length during the first trimester of pregnancy, numerous studies also analyze cervical length during the third trimester of pregnancy to evaluate the risk of preterm birth, but mostly to forecast the time of delivery.

Regarding the correlation of cervical length during the third trimester of pregnancy with preterm delivery, in a study of Papastefanou in 1180 low-risk singleton pregnancies cervical length was measured by ultrasound at 24–30 weeks of gestation. It was found that 0.85% of the study population had preterm birth before 34 weeks of gestation and 5.08% had preterm birth before 37 weeks of gestation. Cervical length in the first group of women who had preterm labor before 34 weeks was shorter (mean 11 mm, $p < 0.001$) than the cervical length of women who gave birth after 34 weeks of gestation (mean cervical length 31 mm). Cervical length was also presented in this study as shorter in the women who had premature birth after 34 but before 37 weeks of gestation (mean cervical length 22 mm, $p < 0.001$) compared to women who eventually gave birth after 37 weeks of gestation (average 31 mm). Thus, it was found that cervical length could predict preterm labor before 34 weeks with a sensitivity of 70% and labor after 34 weeks but below 37 weeks of pregnancy with a sensitivity of 38.3% [34, 54–60]. In another study by Mahmut Kuntay Kokanali, cervical length was measured using transvaginal ultrasound at 34 weeks of gestation in 318 low-risk for preterm birth primiparous women. It was concluded that there was a statistically significant correlation between cervical length at 34 weeks of gestation with the week of gestation that birth took place ($r = 0.614$, $p < 0.001$). After statistical analysis, it was found that cervical length below 25.5 mm predicted preterm labor over 34 weeks but below 37 weeks with 80% sensitivity, specificity of 93.9%, positive predictive value of 52.6%, and a negative predictive value of 98.2%, while a cervical length above 42.5 mm at 34 weeks of gestation predicted an extension of pregnancy after 41 weeks with 70.4% sensitivity, 93.5% specificity, positive 50% predictive value and 97.1% negative predictive value [58–62]. Regarding the prediction of the successful outcome of labor induction by assessment of cervical length during the third trimester of pregnancy, there are several studies examining this relationship. In one of these studies, Hatfield did not document the use of cervical length as an effective predictor of labor induction success. This review included 20 studies of 3101 women who were about to undergo labor induction and who were subjected to cervical length ultrasonographic assessment before the induction. It was found that cervical length predicted successful labor induction outcome (positive predictive value 1.66, 95% CI 1.20–2.31) as well as failure to induction (negative predictive value 0.51, 95% CI 0.39–0.67) [58–62].

Another systematic review of Saccone's used five 735 singleton pregnancy studies to draw conclusions about the importance of cervical length in predicting the timing of spontaneous birth. It was therefore found that a cervical length of less than 30 mm could predict the automatic start of birth within the following week of the cervical length measurement with 64% sensitivity and 60% specificity. Thus, a woman at term pregnancy and with a cervical length of 30 mm has a less than 50% chance of giving birth within the next 7 days, while a woman with a cervical length of 10 mm has a greater than 85% chance of giving birth within the next 7 days of the measurement. Finally, another systematic review of Verhoeven's used 31 studies of 5029 women to record cervical length and labor outcome. It was found that cervical length predicted cesarean section with sensitivity ranging from 14% to 92% and specificity from 35% to 100%. In particular, cesarean section could be predicted at a cervical length of 20 mm with a sensitivity of 82% and a specificity of 34%, at a cervical length of 30 mm with a sensitivity of 0.64 and a specificity of 0.74%, and at a cervical length of 40 mm with a sensitivity of 13% and specificity of 95% [62–66]. According to the literature, there are many ambiguous and contradictory opinions.

However, in our center, Department of Obstetrics and Gynecology of the Democritus University of Thrace Cervical cerclage is performed at a cervical length shorter than 15 mm. In other cases, at a cervical length greater than 15 mm, pessary is recommended for the pregnant woman. In some cases where, despite the cervix cerclage, a shortening of the cervix is observed, a combination of circumcision and pesso is recommended. In all pregnant women at risk of premature delivery, it is recommended administration of progesterone.

In conclusion, preterm birth continues to complicate 11–12% of all pregnancies with a slightly increasing trend in recent years, which is only partially attributable to the increased number of multiple pregnancies. The impact of preterm birth on public health is very serious as it accounts for 70% of neonatal mortality and 50% of neurodevelopmental problems, and based on the results of this study we conclude that the contribution of transvaginal ultrasound during pregnancy in the early recognition of pregnancies at increased risk for preterm birth is significant.

Author details

Panagiotis Tsikouras*, Triada Charmanidou, Stefani Filiou, Georgios Iatrakis, Anastasia Bothou, Efthimios Oikonomou, Dimitrios Kyriakou, Aise Chatzi Ismail Mouchterem, Alexios Alexiou, Konstantinos Nikolettos, Nektaria Kritsotaki, Theopi Nalbanti and Nikolaos Nikolettos
Department of Obstetrics and Gynecology, Democritus University of Thrace, Greece

*Address all correspondence to: tsikouraspanagiotis@gmail.com

References

[1] Elias C, Nogueira PJ, Sousa P. Preterm birth characteristics and outcomes in Portugal, between 2010 and 2018-A cross-sectional sequential study. Health Science Reports. 2023;**6**(2):e1054. DOI: 10.1002/hsr2.1054. eCollection 2023 Feb

[2] Zhu XZ, Deng ZM, Dai FF, Liu H, Cheng YX. The impact of early pregnancy metabolic disorders on pregnancy outcome and the specific mechanism. European Journal of Medical Research. 2023;**28**(1):197

[3] Murray-Davis B, Berger H, Melamed N, Hasan H, Mawjee K, Syed M, et al. Weight gain during pregnancy: Does the antenatal care provider make a difference? A retrospective cohort study. Diabetes, Obesity and Hypertension in Pregnancy Research Network and Southern Ontario Obstetrical Network investigators. CMAJ Open. 2019;**7**(2)

[4] Romero R, Espinoza J, Erez O, Hassan S. The role of cervical cerclage in obstetric practice: Can the patient who could benefit from this procedure be identified? American Journal of Obstetrics and Gynecology. 2006;**194**(1):1-9

[5] Silva TV, Borovac-Pinheiro A, Cecatti JG, Mol BW, et al. Association between cervical length and gestational age at birth in singleton pregnancies: A multicentric prospective cohort study in the Brazilian population. Reproductive Health. 2023;**20**(1):47

[6] Jafari-Dehkordi E, Adibi A, Sirus M. Reference range of the weekly uterine cervical length at 8 to 38 weeks of gestation in the center of Iran. Advanced Biomedical Research. 2015;**4**:115. DOI: 10.4103/2277-9175.157839

[7] Norman JE, Marlow N, Messow CM, Shennan A, Bennett PR, et al. Does progesterone prophylaxis to prevent preterm labour improve outcome? A randomised double-blind placebo-controlled trial (OPPTIMUM). Health Technology Assessment. 2018;**22**(35):1-304

[8] Ashoush S, ElKady O, AlHawwary G. The value of oral micronized progesterone in the prevention of recurrent spontaneous preterm birth: A randomized controlled trial. Acta Obstetricia et Gynecologica Scandinavica. 2017;**96**:1460-1466

[9] Wagh GN, Kundavi Shankar KM, Bachani S. A review of conventional and sustained-release formulations of oral natural micronized progesterone in obstetric indications. Drugs Context. 13 Oct 2021;**10**:2021-7-1. DOI: 10.7573/dic.2021-7-1. eCollection 2021. PMID: 34721615

[10] Romero R, Nicolaides KH, Conde-Agudelo A, O'Brien JM, Cetingoz E, Da Fonseca E, et al. Vaginal progesterone decreases preterm birth ≤ 34 weeks of gestation in women with a singleton pregnancy and a short cervix: An updated meta-analysis including data from the OPPTIMUM study. Ultrasound in Obstetrics & Gynecology. 2016;**48**(3):308-317

[11] Berger R, Abele H, Bahlmann F, Bedei I, Doubek K, Ursula Felderhoff-Müser Prevention and Therapy of Preterm Birth. Guideline of the DGGG, OEGGG and SGGG (S2k Level, AWMF Registry Number 015/025, February 2019) - Part 1 with recommendations on the epidemiology, etiology, prediction. Primary and Secondary Prevention of Preterm Birth Geburtshilfe Frauenheilkd. 2019;**79**(8):800-812.

DOI: 10.1055/a-0903-2671. Epub 2019 Aug 12

[12] Preterm birth aetiology 2004-2008. Maternal factors associated with theHenderson JJ, OA MW, Newnham JP, Pennell CE. e phenotypes: Spontaneous preterm labour, preterm pre-labour rupture of membranes and medically indicated preterm birth. Journal of Maternal-Fetal and Neonatal Medicine. 2012;**25**(6):642-647

[13] Glover AV, Manuck TA. Screening for spontaneous preterm birth and resultant therapies to reduce neonatal morbidity and mortality: A review. Seminars in Fetal & Neonatal Medicine. 2018;**23**(2):126-132

[14] Glover AV, Manuck TA. Screening for spontaneous preterm birth and resultant therapies to reduce neonatal morbidity and mortality: A review. Seminars in Fetal & Neonatal Medicine. 2018;**23**(2):126-132

[15] Jwala S, Tran TL, Terenna C, McGregor A, Andrel J, Leiby BE, et al. Evaluation of additive effect of quantitative fetal fibronectin to cervical length for prediction of spontaneous preterm birth among asymptomatic low-risk women. Journal of Maternal-fetal & Neonatal Medicine. 2016;**95**(8):948-955

[16] Newnham JP, White SW, Meharry S, Lee HS, Pedretti MK, Arrese CA, et al. Reducing preterm birth by a statewide multifaceted program: An implementation study. American Journal of Obstetrics and Gynecology. 2017;**216**(5):434-442

[17] Norman JE, Marlow N, Messow CM, Shennan A, Bennett PR, Thornton S, et al. Vaginal progesterone prophylaxis for preterm birth (the OPPTIMUM study): A multicentre, randomised, double-blind trial. Lancet. 2016;**387**(10033):2106-2116

[18] Parra-Saavedra M, Gómez L, Barrero A, Parra G, Vergara F, Navarro E. Prediction of preterm birth using the cervical consistency index. Ultrasound in Obstetrics & Gynecology. 2011;**38**(1):44-51

[19] Suhag A, Berghella V. Cervical cerclage. Clinical Obstetrics and Gynecology. 2014;**57**(3):557-567

[20] Hezelgrave NL, Watson HA, Ridout A, Diab F, et al. Rationale and design of SuPPoRT: A multi-centre randomised controlled trial to compare three treatments: Cervical cerclage, cervical pessary and vaginal progesterone, for the prevention of preterm birth in women who develop a short cervix. BMC Pregnancy and Childbirth. 2016;**16**:358

[21] Goya M, Pratcorona L, Merced C, Rodó C, Valle L, Romero A, et al. Cervical pessary in pregnant women with a short cervix (PECEP): An open-label randomised controlled trial. Lancet. 2012;**379**(9828):1800-1806

[22] Abdel-Aleem H, Shaaban OM, Abdel-Aleem MA. Cervical pessary for preventing preterm birth. Cochrane Database of Systematic Review. 31 May 2013;**2013**(5):CD007873. DOI: 10.1002/14651858.CD007873.pub3. PMID: 23728668

[23] Abdel-Aleem H, Shaaban OM, Abdel-Aleem MA, Aboelfadle Mohamed A. Cervical pessary for preventing preterm birth in singleton pregnancies. Cochrane Database of Systematic Review. 1 Dec 2022;**12**(12):CD014508. DOI: 10.1002/14651858.CD014508. PMID: 36453699

[24] Wennerholm UB, Bergman L, Kuusela P, Ljungström E, Möller AC, Hongslo Vala C, et al. Progesterone, cerclage, pessary, or acetylsalicylic acid for prevention of preterm birth in singleton and multifetal pregnancies—A systematic review and meta-analyses. Frontiers in Medicine. 2023;**10**:1111315. DOI: 10.3389/fmed.2023.1111315

[25] Conde-Agudelo A, Romero R, Da Fonseca E, O'Brien JM, Cetingoz E, Creasy GW, et al. Vaginal progesterone is as effective as cervical cerclage to prevent preterm birth in women with a singleton gestation, previous spontaneous preterm birth, and a short cervix: Updated indirect comparison meta-analysis. American Journal of Obstetrics and Gynecology. 2018;**219**(1):10-25. DOI: 10.1016/j.ajog.2018.03.028

[26] Wolf HM, Romero R, Strauss JF, Hassan SS, Latendresse SJ, Webb BT, et al. Study protocol to quantify the genetic architecture of sonographic cervical length and its relationship to spontaneous preterm birth. BMJ Open. 17 Mar 2022;**12**(3):e053631. DOI: 10.1136/bmjopen-2021-053631. PMID: 35301205

[27] Crane JM, Hutchens D. Transvaginal sonographic measurement of cervical length to predict preterm birth in asymptomatic women at increased risk: A systematic review. Ultrasound in Obstetrics & Gynecology. 2008;**31**(5): 579-587. DOI: 10.1002/uog.5323

[28] Jafari-Dehkordi E, Adibi A, Sirus M. Reference range of the weekly uterine cervical length at 8 to 38 weeks of gestation in the center of Iran. Advanced Biomedical Research. 2015;**4**:115. DOI: 10.4103/2277-9175.157839

[29] Romero R, Espinoza J, Erez O, Hassan S. The role of cervical cerclage in obstetric practice: Can the patient who could benefit from this procedure be identified? American Journal of Obstetrics and Gynecology. 2006;**194**(1):1-9. DOI: 10.1016/j.ajog.2005.12.002

[30] Sperling L, Kiil C, Larsen LU, Qvist I, Bach D, Wøjdemann K, et al. How to identify twins at low risk of spontaneous preterm delivery. Ultrasound in Obstetrics & Gynecology. 2005;**26**(2):138-144

[31] Combs C, Schuit E, Caritis S, Lim A, Garite T, Maurel K, et al. 17-Hydroxyprogesterone caproate in triplet pregnancy: An individual patient data meta-analysis. Global Obstetrics Network (GONet) collaboration. BJOG. 2016;**123**:682-690

[32] Bernasko J, Lee R, Pagano M, Kohn NJ. Is routine prophylactic cervical cerclage associated with significant prolongation of triplet gestation? Journal of Maternal-Fetal and Neonatal Medicine. 2006;**19**:575-578

[33] Young C, Stanisic T, Wynn L, Shrivastava V, Haydon M, Wing D. Use of cerclage in triplet pregnancies with an asymptomatic short cervix. Journal of Ultrasound in Medicine. 2014;**33**:343-347

[34] Papastefanou I, Pilalis A, Eleftheriades M, Souka AP. Prediction of preterm delivery by late cervical length measurement after 24 weeks. Fetal Diagnosis and Therapy. 2015;**38**(3):200-204

[35] Navathe R, Saccone G, Villani M, Knapp J, Cruz Y, Boelig R, et al. Decrease in the incidence of threatened preterm labor after implementation of transvaginal ultrasound cervical length universal screening. Journal of Maternal-Fetal & Neonatal Medicine. 2019;**32**(11):1853-1858

[36] Kehila M, Abouda HS, Sahbi K, Cheour H, Chanoufi MB. Ultrasound cervical length measurement in prediction of labor induction outcome. Journal of Neonatal-Perinatal Medicine. 2016;**9**(2):127-131

[37] Léhner G, Reif P, Avian A, Kollmann M, Lakovschek IC, Lang U, et al. Does third trimester cervical length predict duration of first stage of labor? Wiener klinische Wochenschrift. 2019;**131**(19-20):468-474

[38] Williams JE, Pugh Y. The late preterm: A population at risk. Critical Care Nursing Clinics of North America. 2018;**30**(4):431-443. DOI: 10.1016/j.cnc.2018.07.001. Epub 2018 Oct 16

[39] Johnston KM, Gooch K, Korol E, Vo P, Eyawo O, Bradt P, et al. The economic burden of prematurity in Canada. BMC Pediatrics. 2014;**14**:93

[40] Hansen A, Moloney ME, Cockerham-Morris C, Li J, Chavan NR. Preterm birth prevention in Appalachian Kentucky: Understanding barriers and facilitators related to transvaginal ultrasound cervical length surveillance among prenatal care providers. Womens Health Report (New Rochelle). 2020;**1**(1):293-300

[41] Vafaei H, Rahimirad N, Hosseini SM, Kasraeian M, Asadi N, Raeisi Shahraki H, et al. Triage by cervical length sonographic measurements for targeted therapy in threatened preterm labor: A double blind randomized clinical trial. International Journal of Reproductive BioMedicine. 2017;**15**(11):697-702

[42] Goldstein MJ, Bailer JM, Gonzalez-Brown VM. Uterocervical angle in predicting spontaneous preterm birth: A systematic review and meta-analysis. AJOG Global Reports. 2023;**3**(3):100240

[43] Nguyen THT, Vu VT, Nguyen VQH. Distribution of uterocervical angles of pregnant women at 16^{+0} to 23^{+6} weeks gestation with low risk for preterm birth: First vietnamese cohort of women with singleton pregnancies. BMC Pregnancy Childbirth. 2023;**23**(1):301

[44] Tsikouras P, Galazios G, Zalvanos A, Bouzaki A, Athanasiadis A. Transvaginal sonographic assessment of the cervix and preterm labor. Clinical and Experimental Obstetrics & Gynecology. 2007;**34**(3):159-162

[45] van de Mheen, Schuit E, Lim AC, Porath MM, Papatsonis D, Erwich JJ, et al. Prediction of preterm birth in multiple pregnancies: Development of a multivariable model including cervical length measurement at 16 to 21 weeks' gestation. Journal of Obstetrics and Gynaecology Canada. 2014;**36**(4):309-319

[46] van de Mheen L, Ravelli AC, Oudijk MA, Bijvank SN, Porath MM, Duvekot JJ, et al. Prediction of time to delivery week-by-week in women with a triplet pregnancy. American Journal of Perinatology. 2016;**33**(14):1394-1400

[47] Tsikouras P, Anastasopoulos G, Bothou A, Chalkidou A, Iatrakis G, Zervoudis S, et al. Comparative evaluation of Arabin pessary and cervical cerclage for the prevention of preterm labor in asymptomatic women with high risk factors. International Journal of Environmental Research and Public Health. 2018;**15**(4):791. DOI: 10.3390/ijerph15040791

[48] Rahman RA, Atan IK, Ali A, Kalok AM, Ismail NAM, Mahdy ZA, et al. Use of the Arabin pessary in women at high risk for preterm birth: Long-term experience at a single tertiary center in Malaysia. BMC Pregnancy Childbirth. 2021;**21**(1):368

[49] Pils S, Springer S, Wehrmann V, Chalubinski K, Ott J. Cervical length dynamics in triplet pregnancies: A retrospective cohort study. Archives of Gynecology and Obstetrics. 2017;**296**(2):191-198

[50] Hiersch L, Rosen H, Okby R, Freeman H, Barrett J, Melamed N. The greater risk of preterm birth in triplets is mirrored by a more rapid cervical shortening along gestation. American Journal of Obstetrics and Gynecology. 2016;**215**(3):357.e1-357.e6

[51] Sananes N, Meyer N, Gaudineau A, Aissi G, Boudier E, Fritz G, et al. Prediction of spontaneous preterm delivery in the first trimester of pregnancy. European Journal of Obstetrics, Gynecology, and Reproductive Biology. 2013;**171**(1):18-22

[52] Kokanali MK, Çelik H, Kokanali D, Taşçi Y. Predictive role of transvaginal ultrasonographic measurement of cervical length at 34 weeks for late pre-term and late-term deliveries in nulliparous women. The Journal of Maternal-Fetal & Neonatal Medicine. 2016;**29**:11

[53] Collins A, Shennan A. A clinical opinion on how to manage the risk of preterm birth in twins based on literature review. The Journal of Maternal-Fetal & Neonatal Medicine. 2016;**29**:1125-1130

[54] Yamasmit W, Chaithong-wongwatthana S, Tolosa JE, Limponqsanurak S, Pereira L, Lumbiganon P. Prophylactic oral betamimetics for reducing preterm birth in women with a twin pregnancy. Cochrane Database of Systematic Reviews. 2015;**8**:CD004733

[55] Crowther CA, Brown J, McKinlay CJD, Middleton P. Magnesium sulphate for preventing preterm birth in threatened preterm labour. Cochrane Database of Systematic Reviews. 2014;**8**:1-89

[56] Bibbo C, Deluca L, Gibbs K, et al. Rescue corticosteroids in twin pregnancies and short term neonatal outcomes. BJOG. 2013;**120**:58-63

[57] Berghella V, Szychowski JM, Owen J, Hankins G, Iams JD, et al. Suture type and ultrasound-indicated cerclage efficacy. Vaginal Ultrasound Trial Consortium. The Journal of Maternal-Fetal & Neonatal Medicine. 2012;**25**:2287-2290

[58] Berghella V, Szychowski JM, et al. Suture type and ultrasound-indicated cerclage efficacy. The Journal of Maternal-Fetal & Neonatal Medicine. 2012;**25**:2287-2290

[59] Berghella V, Ludmir J, Simonazzi G, et al. Transvaginal cervical cerclage: Evidence for perioperative management strategies. American Journal of Obstetrics and Gynecology. 2013;**209**:181-192

[60] Senat MV, Porcher R, Winer N, et al. Prevention of preterm delivery by 17 alpha-hydroxyprogesterone caproate in asymptomatic twin pregnancies with a short cervix: A randomized controlled trial. American Journal of Obstetrics and Gynecology. 2013;**208**(194):e1-e8

[61] Schuit E, Stock S, Rode L, et al. Effectiveness of progestogens to improve perinatal outcome in twin pregnancies: An individual participant data meta-analysis. BJOG: An International Journal of Obstetrics & Gynaecology. 2014;**122**:27-37

[62] Serra V. Increased doses of vaginal progesterone for the prevention of preterm birth in twin pregnancies: A randomised controlled double-blind

multi-Centre trial. BJOG: An International Journal of Obstetrics and Gynecology. 2013;**1**:50-57

[63] Ivandic J, Care A, Goodfellow L, et al. Cervical pessary for short cervix in high risk pregnant women: 5 years experience in a single centre. The Journal of Maternal-Fetal & Neonatal Medicine. Apr 2020;**33**(8):1370-1376. DOI: 10.1080/14767058.2018.1519018. Epub 2018 Sep 25. PMID: 30173599

[64] Mhkow Goya M, Pratcorona L, Merced C, et al. Cervical pessary in pregnant women with a short cervix (PECEP): An open-label randomised controlled trial. Lancet. 2012;**379**:1800-1806

[65] Liem S, Schuit E, Bais J, et al. Pessaries in multiple pregnancy as a prevention of preterm birth (ProTWIN): A randomized controlled trial. American Journal of Obstetrics and Gynecology. 2013;**208**:S

[66] Jarde A, Lewis-Mikhael AM, Dodd JM, et al. The more, the better?, Combining interventions to prevent preterm birth in women at risk: A systematic review and meta-analysis. JOGC. 2017;**39**:1192-1202

Chapter 2

Abnormal Cervical Remodeling Early Depiction by Ultrasound Elastography: Potential Opportunities for Preterm Birth Prevention and Delay

Manuela Cristina Russu, Adriana Elena Ghelmene, Ruxandra Viorica Stănculescu and Şerban Nastasia

Abstract

Early depiction of abnormal cervical remodeling (CR) is a prime information source with days/even weeks to uterine contractions for preterm birth (PTB) risks. CR phases, softening-ripening-dilation, are distinctive by molecular, and timing in preterm/term: integrity loss in ripening and dilation. Changes in extracellular matrix, cellular content, water retention drive progressively to resistance reduction, rising elasticity, relaxing cervical smooth muscle cells (CSMCs) are organized like a sphincter at internal os. Shear Wave Elasticity Imaging-SWEI (dynamic elastography) based on objectively measurable cervical response to deformability is more accurate for early CR depiction from 8–12 weeks vs. conventional ultrasound cervical length (CL) measurements ($16–23^{+6days}$ weeks). SWEI quantifies tissue microstructure, constant fractional stiffness reduction (~ 4%/week), and spatial gradient in Shear Wave Speed (SWS) along cervix, and CL serial measurements in addition offers better strategies for prolongation, actual/future fetal safety, when cervical softness/shortness progresses. Vaginal progesterone (P_4) from early pregnancy to complete 37 weeks is preventive: controls CR, indicated by SWS prior to CL < 25 mm, and cerclage (1–2 stiches) and/or pessary needs, adjuvant to cerclage, for CL < 15 mm after cerclage. Meta-analyses, systematic reviews proved P_4 efficacy in prolongation (>28, 34, 37 weeks) in asymptomatic cases, with characteristic history/actual abnormal CR/shortness, a small better efficacy for vaginal P_4, and cerclage vs. pessary, when separately analyzed; few retrospective studies exist on triple association efficacy for PTB prevention/delay and neonatal outcomes.

Keywords: cervical softening/ripening, human cervical smooth muscle cells, dynamic elastography—Shear Wave Elasticity Imaging, ultrasound, preterm birth, vaginal progesterone, cerclage, pessary

1. Introduction

Cervix uteri is a metabolic active organ, a "gate keeper" in normal pregnancy, an early information prime source about spontaneous preterm birth (sPTB) risks [1], besides other two pathological conditions – preterm/premature membrane rupture (PROM), preterm contractions with which cervical insufficiency/incompetence interlinks in the "Preterm Labor Syndrome" [2], which replaced an earlier five ways acting in cascade/separately: uterine cervical support structures compromise acting alone/associated to the myometrial and membranes over-distension, to decidual hemorrhage, to intrauterine infection/inflammation or to precocious endocrine fetal activation (from maternal or fetal stress) [3]. Vink and Feltovich [4] proposed a new paradigm/concept that sPTB three essential elements (cervical remodeling, myometrium activation-preterm labor, decidua-preterm membrane rupture/hemorrhage) are inextricably intertwined, all lead to each other. These factors are considered as a possible "phenotype" for sPTB [4, 5], such as those that start with premature activation of fetal membranes leading to PROM vs. myometrium premature activation leading to preterm labor vs. premature cervical remodeling leading to cervical failure, but 25% of sPTB are not associated to any phenotype [5].

Prematurity rate has not declined over the past 40 years, or a small decline was followed by a new increase, and despite significant medical and management strategies advances, it has a continuous slow rise, with high offspring morbidity and mortality, affecting 14.8 million babies annually worldwide [6]. Management with actual opportunities of assessment and medical/surgical procedures—elective, urgent, and/or emergency, consuming a substantial portion of the health budget [7, 8] is the aim of modern obstetrics/perinatal medicine societies, being imperative to improve medical understanding of normal/abnormal reproductive tissue structure and function, and how these tissues interact at cellular and biochemical level, and to act accordingly. This chapter focuses on cervix uteri involvement for sPTB prediction and prevention/delay through cervical abnormal remodeling identification by non-invasive novel approach imaging techniques.

2. Gestational cervical remodeling

"Cervical remodeling" is the collective term for progressive cervical changes and recovery during pregnancy, labor, and postpartum, involving four overlapping phases: softening, ripening, dilation, and postpartum repair [9]. Clinicians use terms such as *softening, shortening, funneling, effacing,* and *dilating* interchangeably [10] for gestational cervical deformations, representing tissue intrinsic material changes with anatomical transformations. Cervical insufficiency (CI) determined a lot of comments. According to the American College of Obstetricians and Gynecologists [11], it is defined as "painless cervical dilation after the first trimester with subsequent expulsion of the pregnancy in the second trimester, typically before 24 weeks gestation, without contractions or labor, and in the absence of other clear pathology (as bleeding, infection, ruptured membranes)". It was recommended the terminology "premature cervical remodeling" to describe cervical softening, shortening, funneling, and IO dilation, and to retire the anachronistic "cervical insufficiency" [4].

2.1 Cervix uteri microarchitecture

Human cervical structure was established in the 1940s when Danforth D [12] described cervical stroma—a predominantly homogenous, hydrated, collagenous structure between exo and endocervix, which over time made the distinction to the muscular structure of the uterine corpus. Stroma consists of 85–90% extracellular matrix (ECM) that contains tropocollagen, aggregating to form collagen fiber, and bundles network surrounded by a viscous substance of proteoglycans (decorin, biglycan, asporin, osteomodulin and fibromodulin, lumican, and versican), glycosaminoglycans (GAG: sulfated-chondroitin/dermatan/heparan sulfate and non-sulfated: hyaluronan-hyaluronic acid (HA) GAGs), matricellular proteins (thrombospondin 2; tenascin C); adhesion molecules (fibronectin, integrins-α, β or α-β); specific amino-acids—phenylalanine; enzymes [hyaluronidase, matrix metalloproteinases—MMP: -2, -9; lysyl oxidase-like-1 (LOXl-1), involved in ECM transformations], according to their genes, and water [13]. Cells—about 10–15%—are represented by fibroblasts, smooth muscle, glandular, immune, and vascular cells. Fibroblasts synthesize ECM, rich in collagen fibrils (type I—70%, for tensile strength; type III, 30% for elastic properties) as tropocollagen molecules self-assembled into fibrils—a nanoscale rope-like, and elastin, as tropoelastin to form the elastin fibers complex network intertwined with collagen. Collagen bundles are organized in layers, which remodel differently because of independent molecular processes and cause softening and shortening [14, 15]. Collagen content—measured as hydroxyproline, is constant along pregnancy [9]; second-harmonic generation (SHG) microscopy presents collagen preferentially aligned around the canal [16]. The triple helix arrangement allows collagen to cross-link into complex 3-D networks of fibrils, fibers, and bundles that dictate both firmness and mechanical strength during non-pregnant/pregnant states [17]. From Aspden [18] early theory on three zones in cervix structure—**Figure 1A**, actually cervical stroma is considered heterogenic, and collagen network strength depends on the degree and type of collagen cross-links between each collagen microfibril [20, 21]. Recent studies show significant collagen cross-link heterogeneity in internal OS (IO) compared to external OS (EO) [22]; IO area is the most exposed to stretch, and it is resistant to tension associated with uterine content (fetus, placenta, amniotic fluid), cervical angle in pelvis [10], and fetal membranes properties, their stiffness sustaining IO closure,

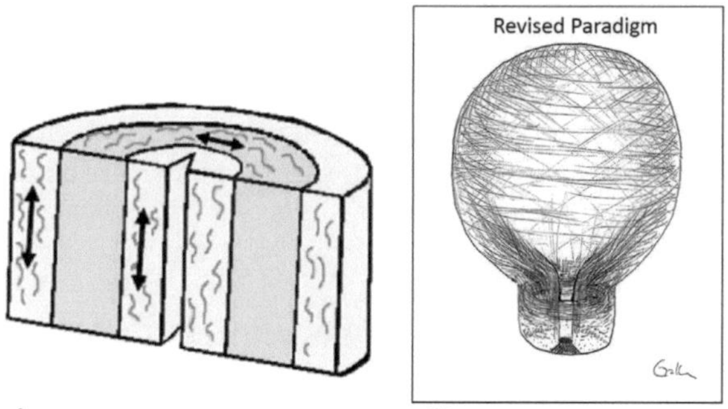

A. B.

Figure 1.
A. The three zone in cervix early theory. B. New paradigm on SMCs at upper cervix half, circumferentially to IO, is like a specialized sphincter; it is not a homogenous collagenous structure, with minimal cellular content, as old paradigm. Adapted from Vink and Myers [19], free PMC article. HHS Public access.

as 3D MRI revealed [23]. Elastin is a high thermal stable protein with an 80-year half-life and a linear, compliant mechanical response to tension, permitting cervix restoration after an applied stretch. Elastic fibers are present mostly in the subepithelial stroma, aligned at early pregnancy as collagen fibers, and undergo structural changes, becoming thicker, shorter, and losing directionality [24, 25]. Proteoglycans have key roles in controlling gradients and availability of potent growth factors, chemokines, cytokines, and morphogens, important in tissue's homeostasis, mechanical strength, development, and repair, by their covalent attachment to collagen fibers surface, contributing to fiber optimal formation [26].

From early studies on cervical structure and functions [27–29], immune—staining with smooth muscle cell markers (α-smooth muscle actin, smooth muscle protein 22 calponin) in non-pregnant women <50 years old cervices proved the presence of smooth muscle cells (HCSMCs) surrounding IO, about 50–60% of tissue, like a specialized sphincter, proved by positive contractile activity tests at oxytocin/nifedipine, similar to uterine SMCs. Bundles of cervical smooth muscle cells (CSMCs) are circumferentially oriented around endocervix canal periphery. Human cervical smooth muscle cells (HCSMCs)' density is gradually reduced from the mid cervix to EO (10%), where contraction tests showed less activity. Gap junctions are present in HCSMCs for direct communication with uterine corpus SMCs [4], a cervical active involvement in pregnancy progression, as Pajntar sustained for a long time [28]. Longitudinal muscle fibers are mostly located in cervix's inner part, while circular muscle fibers are mostly in the outer part. Longitudinal muscles can contract, helping cervical dilatation, while circumferential muscle fiber contraction impedes cervical dilatation, keeping the cervix closed." Dynamic cervix" nomination is used when a short cervix appears without uterine contractions or is correlated to uterine fundus pressure [30]. This discovery changed the paradigm on HCSMCs covering cervix first half part, and their role in IO normal closure, or relaxation-inducing "funneling"/"sphincter failure", the first sign of premature cervical remodeling [19, 30], and increases the duration of latent and active phases of labor [31], according to connections of SMCs from uterine cervix and corpus. Similar CSMCs were discovered in female rats during pregnancy, being considered as a continuous muscular layer from the uterine corpus (**Figure 1A** and **B**) [32].

Resident immune cells -neutrophils, eosinophils, and macrophages are present in cervix; their location and relative number change during pregnancy [33, 34]. Rat's cervices pathological exams [35] proved macrophages role in remodeling, mainly in ripening normal/abnormal timing. There are registered reduced cell nuclei density, decreased collagen content and structure, and a greater presence of macrophages per unit area in rats under progesterone receptor antagonist (onapristone/mifepristone) or after ovariectomy on day 17 postbreeding, similar to aspects before term.

2.2 Timing of cervical remodeling

Qualitative and quantitative cervical softness/stiffness and length dynamic changes previous to uterine contractions onset are harboring different mechanisms in term/PTB regarding cervical involvement in "closing"/"opening", to prevent/delay sPTB/to induce labor, were better understood using mathematical or animal models instead of cervical biopsies because women's risks [36], and confounders by variations in timing and collected samples region [37]. Shorter pregnancy duration and mice cervices resistance to break/stretch made mice prone to study [38]. Evidences provided similarity in women, and mice regarding dynamic gestational cervical remodeling [9, 37, 39], and simulations showed that changes are centered on stroma ECM content, which are associated to changes of SMCs surrounding IO [30], and all control gestational tissue's mechanical behavior.

2.2.1 Premature cervical extracellular matrix changes inducing preterm/premature cervical failure

Cervical stroma ensures mechanical properties [40] by ECM molecules arranged in a scaffold/matrix, and cells. One must understand mathematical models through Humphrey and Rajagopal [41] mixture theory. Updated after 20 years [42] for soft tissue growth [changing mass, solid (cells, fibers), and fluid-interstitial], and remodeling (changing microstructure) for adaption at new growth imposed functions. Microarrays and gene analysis [43] in murine models revealed two distinct phases – softening and ripening. Cervical human transcriptome is mentioned more than a decade ago [44], with some considerations on distinct cervical microRNA profiles in women destined to sPTB [45], cervical softening—an active phase, as shown in nearly daily assessment in murine models [15, 39] with rapid onset after conception, is defined as the first measurable increase in tissue distensibility versus to non-pregnant, with a precisely timed activation of slow molecular, microstructural, and mechanical changes up to term/labor [9], regarding cellularity, collagen, elastin, GAGs, proteoglycans, water. Softening drives alterations in collagen fibers organization and alignment, inducing a distinctive arrangement—short, thick, and curved, with low linearity, and change in the number and type of cross-linking between newly formed fibrils, coinciding with a marked increase in hyaluronic acid (HA), and water uptake, globally reducing mechanical resistance to tension [15, 46], an influx/activation of immune cells releasing MMPs degrading ECM [37], increase elasticity, and prepare inferior segment for delivery. Collagen waviness confers tissue isotropy and heterogeneity, destabilizing mechanical integrity with great deformations and relaxations and increased compliance necessary for uterine cavity rising pressure, with tissue integrity maintenance. Ripening—a term used first by Winkler and Rath [47]—is near labor onset, with rapid evolution, cervix marked softening and shortening. Preterm and term cervical changes are similar, not identical; sPTB can result from aberrant events timing [4]. Murine studies showed differences in the molecular mechanisms governing preterm and term ripening [38, 48]. Untimely cervical ripening in early gestation—earlier than normal (before 24–36^6 days weeks, in women), predisposes to CI, responsible for recurrent late miscarriage/sPTB, and cervical ripening inadequate in late pregnancy is associated with induction failure/prolonged labor, possible involvement of EMC and CSMCs from IO [30]. Murine preterm-induced delivery showed a dramatic reduction of mature collagen fibers, increased new fibrils synthesis, packing disorganization by the gradual replacement of mature cross-linked collagen with collagen harboring reduced cross-linking, less cross-linking between fibers of new fibrils of tropocollagen, which are shorter and thicker than in non-pregnant, besides the distinctive arrangement of fibers—from being aligned to curling, becoming isotropic [46], greater spaces between fibers, decline in thrombospondin-2 and tenascin-C [36], and ECM high hydration [49], the parallelism between water and hyaluronic acid (HA) with very hydrophilic large molecular weight-hyaluronan, increases wet weight vs. controls, and in mice at term [36, 43], affecting collagen organization [50]. The interstitial fluid controls tissue stiffness response, water content increases by 5%, modifying cervix mechanical properties, generating an unbalance/non-equilibrium state [51], and the untimed ripening initiates rapid incremental

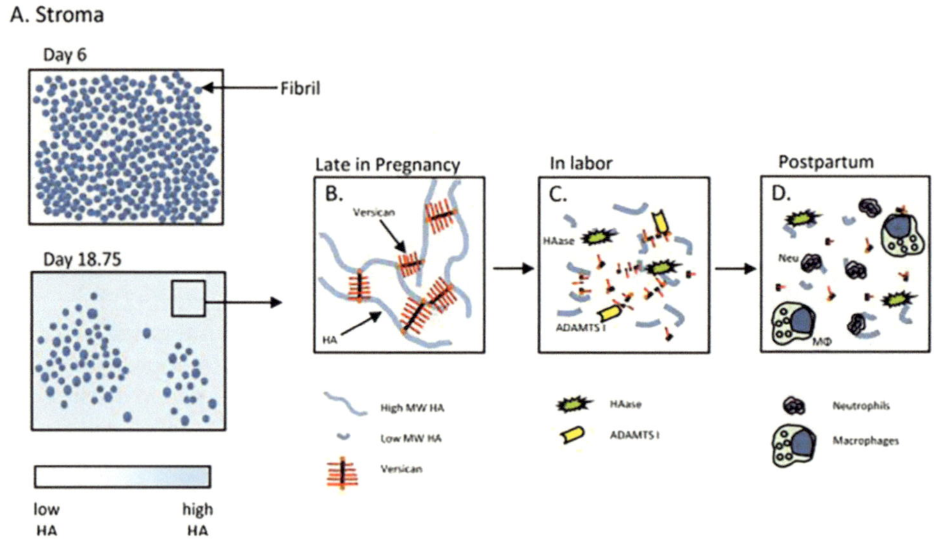

Figure 2.
Proposed model for mice cervical remodeling for mechanical resistance reduce. A. Increase of high molecular weight (MW) hyaluronan in ECM from early to late pregnancy. B. At pregnancy end, high levels HA and versican form cross-links, which are associated with water uptake, increased tissue compliance, visco-elasticity, and collagen disorganization. C. During labor, enzymes (hyaluronidase and ADAMTS enzymes) cleave HA, and versican, causing cervical tissue integrity and complete loss for dilation. D. During postpartum repair, low MW hyaluronan, versican fragments, and damaged collagen are removed by immune cells—neutrophils and macrophages. Adapted from Timmons et al. [15]. PMC free article. HHS Public access.

fall in cervical mechanical strength (**Figure 2**) [37]. As in other tissues (cartilage and blood vessels) with complex mechanical behavior, the relative ratio of collagen to proteoglycans is an important determinant of cervix visco-elasticity, compliance, and ultimate function [52].

The first presented 3D anisotropic hyperelastic model [38], based on Langevin statistical mechanics for human and mice gestational mechanical response, revealed: constant total collagen content per volume along pregnancy; mature collagen cross-link disorganization in human ripening cervix evolves by an increase in tissue acid solubility, along pregnancy; mice collagen cross-link disorganization progresses from d6 (when bundles are larger) to d15, with little change after d15. This difference explains mouse cervix resistance to break in uniaxial tensile test compared to human, in non-pregnant and pregnant state.

The stiffness progressive reduction in normal human pregnancies starts from first trimester (>2 vs. non-pregnant). It continues in the second, but not between the second and third trimester, with consistent recovery after delivery, to the level of early pregnancy, as ectocervix aspiration technique depicted [53]. Cervical shortening normally starts from mid-pregnancy and progresses until delivery, as ultrasound longitudinal studies on cervix length (CL) sustain [54], being a normal 30 mm CL at pregnancy beginning, with individual variations, from population, age, parity, and gestational outcomes, as a systematic review, and meta-analysis report [55].

EMC organization and composition aberrant regulation during softening, a tissue property, may contribute to premature shortening—a tissue deformation that results from an evolving 3D stress state, and the intrinsic constituents remodeling [56], softening plus shortening being considered as dysfunctional EMC remodeling [20], and IO "funneling" is next step, due to softness, and sphincterian HCSMCs relaxation

[30], added to dysfunctional remodeling that starts invariably from IO [57], where is the higher stress compared to EO. EO is not significantly loaded until the cervix has significantly shortened [58], and 3D hyperelastic anisotropic model, revealed relative similar stress to both orifices, and the middle part is between those in the IO and EO [38].

2.2.2 Premature relaxation of cervical smooth muscles cells promoting preterm/premature cervical failure

One offers special attention on HCSMCs presence as a circumferential sphincter at IO level, since the new paradigm on their role in cervical closure in normal pregnancy [30]. A smooth muscle sphincter at IO, is considered one of the most important anatomic structures for pregnancy's normal progression, when it is contracted [10], and its relaxation is associated with the onset of labor, as it was supposed [59]. From Leppert [60] early studies, one knows that in early pregnancy, fibroblasts and CSMCs proliferation is at the highest level and decreases progressively, whereas apoptosis increases progressively in later pregnancy, parallel to water content in interstitial tissue, inducing mechanical imbalance [51]. Cervical contractile function contributes to cervix stiffness and closure maintenance until the latter part of the third trimester. During the ripening and dilation phases, the HCSMCs are not just a passive responder to uterine contractions; they independently initiate their own contractions, and biochemically their stretch increases MMPs [61], and proinflammatory cytokine secretions [62], representing new mechanisms on premature CR, and possible failure. Vink et al. [63] proved in pregnant women cervices with premature cervical failure (PCF) that CSMCs defect of contractility, and reduced IO sphincter tonus appear when CSMCs are exposed to a soft ECM. It is suggested that a soft ECM may lead to decreased CSMCs contractility and IO sphincter laxity, so ECM rigidity modulates HCSMCs contractility.

HCSMCs are physiological modulated by hormones (estrogens, progesterone, and oxytocin—increases intracellular calcium levels), local paracrine signals (inflammatory chemokines and cytokines), extracellular vesicles (exosomes and ectosomes), and pharmacological agents used for cervical ripening and labor induction. Vink et al. [64] demonstrated that E2 increases HCSMCs contractility by rising actin contractility, and calcium levels—less than oxytocin, and favors pregnancy progression, and

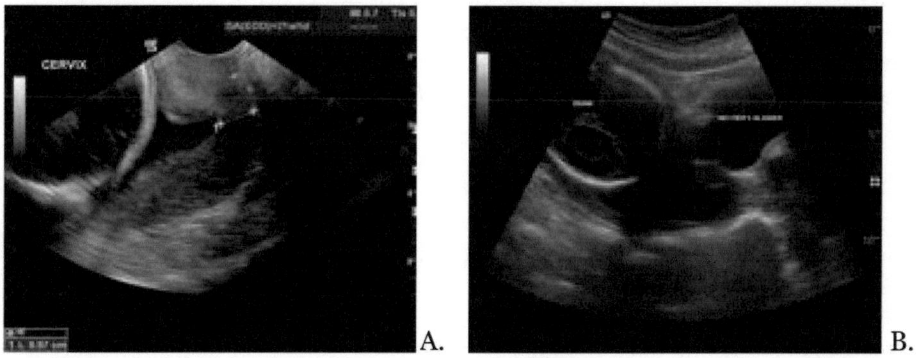

Figure 3.
A: funneling of IO, with shape of T, Y, V, or the most dangerous of U, associated to short cervix (between white markers) B: complete cervical effacement (authors proper archive: [65]).

P_4 reduces HCSMCs contractility, by oxytocin-induced contractility alterations, and intracellular calcium flux; P_4 appears favorable for IO "funneling"/dilation.

Since many years of conventional/standard sonography, starting from 16th weeks gestation, may show shortness and funneling, **Figure 3**. Funneling is considered more predictive than shortness to PTB risk, and it imposes a cervical stitch [64, 66]. Sludge association with short cervix (<25 mm) increases sPTB risks [67].

3. Hypothesis and realities on gestational cervical remodeling timing: molecular insights

Two mouse models have provided new insights into distinct processes of preterm CR: infectious/inflammatory model [68, 69] and progesterone loss/withdrawn/non-infectious model, with differences in gene pathways in preterm, and term. Analyzes of preterm mice collagen structure changes [36] showed that immune pathways system activation is sufficient but not necessary for premature ripening [33, 37, 43, 48] being differences regarding collagen fibers in preterm P_4 withdrawn/mifepristone-induced, infected-induced, and term ripening.

3.1 Inflammation in premature cervical ripening

Lipopolysaccharide (LPS) administration in amniotic sac surroundings elicits a proinflammatory response similar to infection, preterm labor progressing without P_4 concentration loss in circulation several hours after administration [68]. SHG demonstrated an interfibrillar spacing increase in collagen fibrils, with increased pores lacking collagen signal in SHG, when LPS treated mice, and preferential disruption collagen fiber architecture in the subepithelial region compared to mid-stroma region, and neutrophils infiltration. Rodents models demonstrated that ripening may be characterized as a physiologic inflammatory process, by myeloid immune cells, as neutrophils, with their chemotactic factors [69], with a temporal coincidence of decreased density of cell nuclei, decline in cross-linked extracellular collagen, and increased presence of macrophages, sustaining the immune cells hypothesis [70–72], so cervical increased biomechanic distensibility is before uterine contractile capabilities for labor. Flow cytometry and cell sorting were used to determine immune cells role in ECM remodeling before, during, and after parturition. Myeloid immune cells/leukocytes invade EMC and are activated to product proinflammatory mediators [IL-8, monocyte chemo-attractant protein-1 (MCP-1), IL-1β, and TNF-α], and proteolytic enzymes [73] altering EMC. Markers of myeloid cell differentiation and activation were used to define phenotype and function [73]. Peripheral blood does not reflect changes in cervical myeloid cell numbers. The proinflammatory mediators are ripening inducers, through prostaglandins [74], high concentrations of inflammatory cytokines (IL-6, IL-8, and MCP-1) are depicted in human PTB cervix [75]. Monocytes and eosinophils increase in cervix before birth, in a progesterone-regulated fashion, whereas macrophages number is unchanged. The cytologic conclusion is that myeloid-derived cells do not orchestrate processes required for cervical ripening initiation before birth [73].

Macrophages are analyzed in many studies. They are present in gestational cervix with different phenotypes (M1 and M2), considered to be most involved in tissue postpartum repair, sustained by increased mRNA expression of Csfr1, and markers of alternatively activated M2 in labor, or shortly after fetal expulsion [73]. Hunter et al. [34] described a special phenotype of macrophages or phagocytic leukocytes, partially similar with blood—born monocytes, present from the 12th week in normal cases, their absence being a sPTB risk marker. These cells have critical role in cervical immunity, by preventing microbial translocation to feto-placental unit. Leukocyte insufficient recruitment to cervix is supposed to be associated with sPTB recurrence (<34 weeks). The cytokines, and MMPs are increased only in inflammation-induced sPTB, not in term ripening, where is no infection [34].

Prostaglandins are used to induce labor, according to their essential intervention in LPS-mediated preterm ripening, but not term or antiprogestin-driven preterm ripening [76].

Actually, there is a connection between amniotic fluid inflammation and imminent PTB prediction when short cervix in asymptomatic cases, starting with amniotic proteome analysis [77]; inflammation is a giant disruptor of gestational maternal-fetal homeostasis.

3.2 Premature progesterone withdrawn/progesterone receptors loss/ responsiveness in premature cervical ripening

Since 1960, from Cullen and Harkness studies on rat's cervix [78], one knows steroid hormones role in cervical stroma cells specific functions, and complex series of molecular events in pregnancy, and parturition. Steroid hormones actions are proved on HCSMCs surrounding IO [79], through their receptors (ER, PR). Progesterone exerts a dominant role for most of the pregnancy duration to initiate a loss of tissue strength yet maintain competence in the softening phase, which starts early in pregnancy when P_4 is high, E_2 is low, and normal ripening is at the gestation end [9, 80] to permit fetal delivery after active dilation. The reduced P_4/E_2 ratio—a parturition hallmark, begins the cascade of accelerated cervical ripening, responsible for the final structural integrity loss, necessary for fetus safe passage. P_4/E_2 ratio is high during softening; the highest P_4 concentration correlated with the least amount of new collagen fibril synthesis, E2 significantly rising new collagen, and progressively increased levels as P_4 decreases near term, when P_4/E_2 ratio is the lowest [81]. P_4 controls GAGs modulating ECM [82] and counteracts inflammation [83]. The studies on rats [84] showed that PR genomic receptors modulate the transition from a soft to a ripened cervix in term and PTB. Studies on many mammalian species have shown that softening shift to ripening occurs while blood progesterone is near peak concentrations, being discussed as a responsiveness loss to progesterone, a common final mechanism for mammalian cervix remodeling for term birth preparation [70]. P_4 sustains cervical softening and ripening, mediated by a stable stromal cell population, expressing PR-A, and through interactions with resident macrophages, the inflammatory ripening processes are mediated in birth preparation [85]. In ovariectomy-induced systemic progesterone loss, it was not registered hypertrophy, extracellular collagen, or macrophage number changes [35]. Yellon [70] appreciates that the structure and macrophage census in cervix is sufficient for premature ripening and birth before term; PRs are localized on other cells than macrophages, making possible interactions between cells to facilitate the loss of progesterone receptor-mediated actions, as part of a final common mechanism that ripens the cervix in certain preterm etiologies, and in term deliveries.

P_4 non-genomic membrane receptors mechanism is dominant in mice, besides genomic mechanism, mediated by isoform A [85] for prepartum softening and ripening, which start before birth, when systemic P_4 is near peak concentration [72], through stroma fibroblasts, but not macrophages. Smooth muscles, innate immune cells, and mainly pregnancy-activated lymphocytes have P_4 membrane receptors, which fibroblasts are missing. P_4 has immune-modulatory proprieties by the 31 kDa protein "progesterone induced-blocking factor", synthesized by human lymphocytes, which inhibits natural killer cells, and modifies cervical, and decidua cytokines balance. RU486/mifepristone mice administration on the 13th day of gestation induced the onset of preterm labor within several hours [43]. This model presents significant ECM disorganization: more and larger spaces between collagen fibers, higher cervical wet weight, a 5% increased water content *vs* LPS infected mice model, with reduced edema. RU-486 group cervix weight being similar to term cervix. Premature RU-48-induced ripening results from an acceleration of the process, in place during term ripening, as well as partial activation of proinflammatory, and immune-suppressive process, which is observed during normal postpartum repair, different from LPS-induced PTB, where only the neutrophil stroma population is increased, without parallel monocytes, and eosinophils populations, or systemic blood rise; no blood systemic monocytes levels increased in any studied group [43].

Japanese studies on cultured cervical stroma fibroblasts in cases with refractory PCF and recurrent pregnancy loss [86] have a remarkable discovery: namely, cervical fibroblasts' PRs down-regulation, with impairment of P_4 inhibitory effect on lipopolysaccharide-induced inflammatory stimuli, and consecutive PCF. These results suggest that abnormal cervical ripening in CI is caused by down-regulation of P_4 signaling at receptor level and provides a novel insight into the molecular mechanism of PTB.

4. Premature/preterm cervical microstructure remodeling assessment

The current approach to evaluating cervix state relies on digital assess (with Bishop scoring [87], first proposed for labor induction success), subjective appreciation as "soft, medium, hard/firm", and conventional sonographic examination [54] being now compelling evidence that changes in viscoelastic properties are key to cervix function. Cervical length (CL) measurements are suboptimal means to assess early remodeling, providing no data on consistency [88], and because of high negative predictive value, when used as a screening test [89]. Some studies tried to give indirect data on cervical softness during conventional sonography: cervical sliding sign—assessing cervix resistance to gentle probe compression [90], cervical mucus plug distance—part of the plug nearest to vaginal microflora, as an additional sign for CR [91]. One gives much attention to CL value in asymptomatic cases: ≤15 mm before 20 weeks gestation has a dramatic and significantly higher risk of early PTB than at 20–24 weeks [92] and to differences between universal screening and selective screening in conjunction with independent risk factors for a short cervix ≤25 mm at 20–24 weeks [93]: race-ethnicity; current tobacco use; prior indicated preterm birth; a prior cervical excisional procedure. If only women with any of these variables were offered transvaginal CL screening, the specificity would increase from 62.8% for universal screening to 96.5% with a risk-based approach. The sensitivity with one variable present was 62.8%, and with two factors, 14%. The Cochrane Database Systematic Review [94] on the knowledge of CL in singleton pregnancies with symptoms vs. no knowledge up to the year 2018 showed a prolongation with only 4 days before 34 weeks gestation.

4.1 Innovative methods to objectivate premature cervical microstructure remodeling

Non-invasive methods are adopted in maternal-fetal medicine for collagen architecture assessment, clinicians collaborating with biomechanical engineers and other scientists to reveal crucial structural properties changes during pregnancy and labor. Cervical microstructure is a very good objective for new proposed *in vivo* techniques based on quantification of mechanical, optical, or electrical tissue properties: increased hydration with preconceptional collagen organization loss, and/or cervical elasticity [95].

Histopathology is the golden standard for tissue remodeling assessment. Electron/polarized light microscopy, two-photon microscopy, and fluorescence microscopy, with different dyes/antibodies for staining and with limited physicochemical changes on biological tissue, are in trend for slice sizes and collagen content accurate diagnosis. SHG scanning endomicroscopy was proposed to visualize gestational CR in many studies in Europe and the USA. There were recently three accurate collagen fiber extraction techniques (in 3D volume) for quantitative collagen content assessment [96]. SHG permits cervical collagen content longitudinal assessments along pregnancy [12 (first trimester), 23 (second trimester), and 32 (third trimester) gestational weeks], with images archive, and comparison at each visit [97].

Literature mentions numerous new approaches, depending on sites/centers resources and medical staff training, to visualize cervix microstructure: near-infrared spectroscopy and near-infrared Raman microspectroscopy (optical techniques), light-induced fluorescence by callascope—specifically designed to assess cervical ripening, and functions by measuring the natural fluorescence of cervical non-soluble collagen, other methods combine ultrasound to new capabilities to visualize cervix deformability at different levels, by devices intravaginal/intracervical introduced, capturing differences between stiff and soft cervix, as aspiration and cervical consistency index, spectroscopic photo-acoustic imaging (first used in USA, for collagen/water ratio assessment in murine cervices [88], acoustic attenuation; all these methods are not in this subchapter focus.

4.2 Ultrasound-based techniques for cervical microstructure evaluation

Different from conventional ultrasound, various imaging modalities are actually prone to visualize changes in reproductive organs as collagen fibers content and characteristics (density, size, morphology, and orientation/alignment) along pregnancy, and associated to computational tools may quantify, and predict softness abnormal progress, and shift to ripening, before cervical shortness and funneling, in asymptomatic cases, for early sPTB prevention/delay.

4.2.1 B-mode ultrasound elastography: strain/static elastography: shear wave speed estimation elastography/dynamic elastography

Elastography association with conventional/standard ultrasound aimed to bring new data on cervical stiffness, and sPTB, being two types of elastography used in clinical practice: strain elastography-SE (static elastography) and shear wave speed estimation elastography-shear wave speed (SWS) (dynamic elastography).

Strain elastography, a direct biomechanical testing, measures cervix deformation percentage, expressed as a strain value, computer analyzed on a color map (produced by a specialized software), when gentle transducer movements compress a region of interest (ROI: IO, EO, entire cervix [98, 99]) during ordinary B-mode ultrasound vaginal scanning (mid-sagital plan) for CL. Increased strain reflects increased deformation (softer tissue), decreasing strain reflects reduced deformation (stiffer tissue); dichotomous variables are usually constructed to describe whether each patient's measurement is in the bottom quartile (≤25th centile) for each cervical region [98]. The USA results sustained that strain measurements obtained in a cross-sectional view of IO were significantly associated with sPTD (<37 weeks) [98]. The strain values corresponding to 25th centile in IO were 0.19 for the endocervical canal and 0.14 for the entire cervix. Women with strain values ≤25th centile were approximately 80% less likely to subsequently deliver preterm than those whose values were > 25th centile (entire cervix: OR: 0.17; 95% CI: 0.03–0.9; endocervical canal OR: 0.2; 95% CI: 0.03–0.96). Patient's characteristics influence the results (parity, prior preterm deliveries, gestational age at examination, CL, mainly when it is <25 mm [100]).

Despite new real-time quantitative data on cervix morphology and architecture, there are some limitations regarding distance more than 1.5 cm from the transducer, if tissue is inhomogeneous, and if ROI is placed at an angle above 20° from the compression direction; it does not allow quantification of tissue stiffness, when the intensity of force (stress) is unknown, but new devices have press indicator; interobserver variability.

Shear wave speed (SWS)/dynamic shear wave elasticity image (SWEI), can differentiate between soft and firm cervices by measuring ultrasound speed through a tissue: SWS is faster through firm, and slower through soft tissues [101, 102] (**Figure 4**). SWEI assesses women's quantitative stiffness from early (5–14 weeks) to late (40 weeks) gestation, with assessment at EO [104], mid *cervix* (at bladder reflection level), at IO proximity [105], being recognized the depth importance on SWEI estimations in IO, and EO along pregnancy [106]. It is a constant fractional reduction in SWS (average 4%/week), considered the most critical value for birth timing prediction, increasing with gestational age (GA), and a spatial gradient along CL: the most important softness is at the proximal end—9%/week, and 2%/week at distal end [107]. There are differences in SWS reduction reports from first to third trimester: 52% [107], 42% [108], or only a 12% decrease [104], being demonstrated that SWS declines progressively with GA between 18 and 24 weeks, being higher at IO than at EO, at each GA, IO is the best area to assess [103], because collagen fibers longitudinal alignment along endocervical canal, and at it is proximal part, not circumferential as they are near cervix edge, as microscopy revealed on specimens collected at hysterectomy, and reduced by 1.4 at every 10 years of maternal age, not by BMI [109].

Women with a soft cervix were 3.3 times more likely to have a short cervix, and 1.5 times more likely to have had a prior sPTB than cases who did not have a soft cervix compared to a cervix that was neither short nor soft. Softness increases by 1.5 times the risk of repeating sPTB. Prevalence of sPTB is higher by 18 fold <37 weeks, and by 120 fold <34 weeks, when a soft cervix (C) (<25th percentile for GA defined by SWEI at IO) is associated with short C (cut-off <25 mm) compared to normal CL, at 18–24 weeks [103]. Study conclusion was that softness is an independent risk factor for sPTB <37 and < 34 weeks, regardless of shortness presence, or sPTB history. **Table 1** shows the superior specificity and positive likelihood ratio (LR) values for sPTB (<34 and <37 weeks), when softness and shortness are combined.

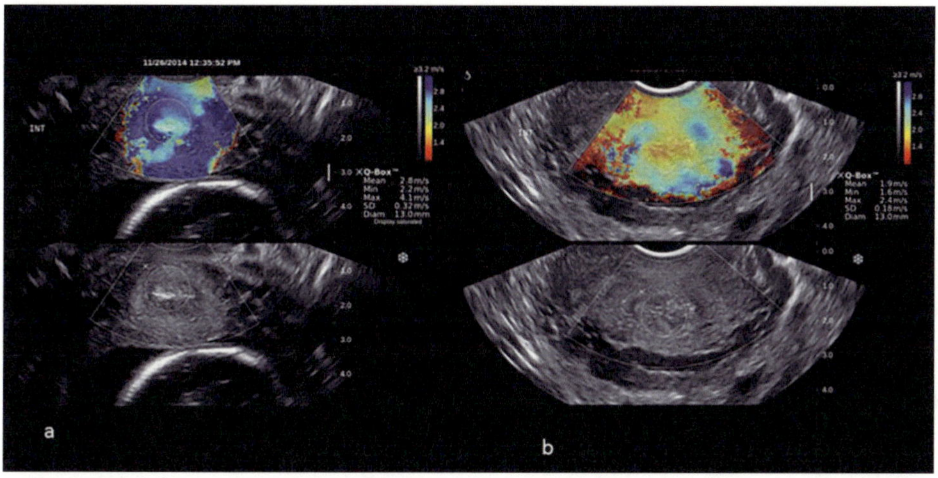

Figure 4.
Shear wave elastography in the cross-sectional planes of the external cervical OS of two patients at 21 weeks of gestation; (a) a non-soft cervix (shear wave speed (SWS) = 2.3 m/s [SWS 25th percentile = 1.72 m/s]); (b) a soft cervix with a SWS of 1.6 m/s (≤25th percentile). High SWS is shown in blue and low SWS in red. Adapted from Hernandez-Andrade et al. [103]. Free PMC article, HHS Public Access.

Sensitivity (%)	Specificity (%)	Positive LR	Negative LR
Softness shortness combination vs. short *cervix* for PTB risks <34 weeks			
33.3/33.3	98.2/96.1	18.5/12.7	0.7/0.7
Softness shortness combination vs. short *cervix* for PTB risk <37 weeks			
19.4/19.4	98.4/96.3	8.5/5.2	0.8/0.8

Table 1.
Sensitivity, specificity, LR for PTB when softness, shortness combination vs. short cervix. Results from Hernandez-Andrade et al. [103].

4.3 Anatomical computer simulation models to study human cervix uteri remodeling

The unanswered questions on premature CR, and sPTB prediction wait for answers from anatomically correct computer simulation models of pregnant human pelvis, uterus, and cervix geometry. The stress/stretch amount on the IO area depends on cervix angle/position in the pelvis [10] and on amniotic membrane strength, assessed by 3D MRI [24]. Vink and Feltovich [4] elaborated on the hypothesis that combining weak membranes to an undesirable cervical position/angle that increases the stretch on IO ultimately leads to cervical dilation and sPTB. The engineering tools will help to evaluate/predict sPTB using computational biomechanics and finite element analysis to study sPTB causes and to develop a diagnosis tool for outcome prediction [110]. One may individualize the computer models (which incorporate patient-specific tissue properties and ultrasound-derived parameters) to predict and/or identify which women with premature CR will deliver preterm.

5. Potential opportunities for preterm birth prevention/delay in preterm cervical changes

Vaginal progesterone, cervical stitch-cerclage, and pessary are actual opportunities to prevent/delay sPTB, when history, and/or current monitoring indicate gestational cervical untimed progressive changes, discussing them separately or comparing the beneficial/harmful effects of two of them cerclage *vs* P_4/pessary, and less all three therapies.

5.1 Progesterone for cervical Remodeling timing and preterm birth prevention

Progesterone works for "quiescence" or "silencing" uterine contractions [111], and exerts a dominant role for most pregnancies to initiate a loss of tissue strength yet maintain competence in softening, and delays ripening onset, maintaining stiffness [103], and CL > 25 mm, as was proved by RCT [112], a meta-analysis [113], and meta-analysis on individual data [114]. A retrospective study on P_4 administration when short cervix <25 mm at 24^{+0} and 33^{+6} weeks gestation revealed P_4 efficacy in pregnancy prolongation after 34 weeks (**Figure 5**) [115].

Natural micronized progesterone vaginal administration (200 mg/capsule, or 90 mg gel), from early pregnancy up to 36^{+6} weeks, induced an sPTB<33 weeks reduction of 38% in singleton and 31% in twins, and for sPTB recurrence in cases with sPTB history [11, 116], and sPTB prophylaxis in cases with short cervix (OPPTIMUM study) [117]. Actual data in twins pregnancy prolongation >34 weeks are contradictory on P_4 beneficial effects [118]. There is only a 0.02% reduction of sPTB absolute risk in singleton, when short cervix [119]. It is important to add that only vaginal P_4 has anti-inflammatory effects on the murine maternal-fetal

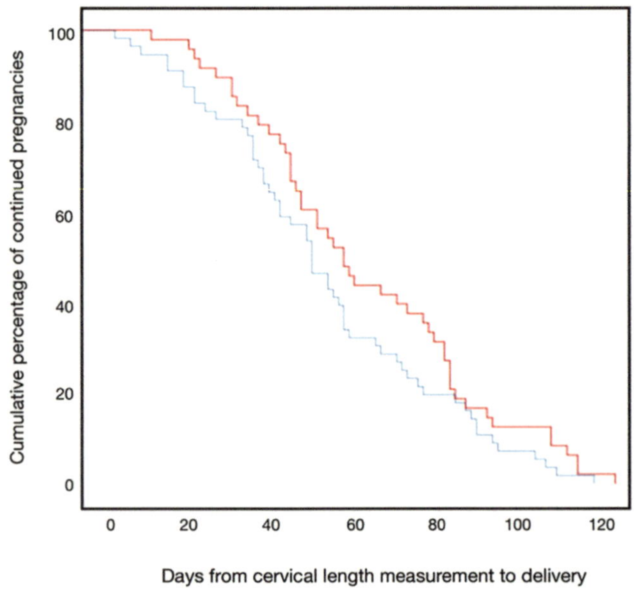

Figure 5.
Kaplan-Meier plot for days to delivery. The Kaplan-Meier plot of delivery by days from cervical length measurement of the progesterone treatment group (red line) and the non-treatment group (blue line). Adapted from Luxenbourg et al. [115]. Free PMC article. HHS Public access.

interface [120, 121], which are absent when comparing weekly i.m. 17α-hydroxyprogesterone caproate to vaginal P_4 for short cervix [122], and has more side effects, FDA does not recommend it since 2022.

Cervical static/strain elastography (with E-cervix™ program) for entire cervix – IO, EO, ECI was proposed to continue cervical strain assessments, together with conventional ultrasound, 1 week after P_4 treatment for CL ≤25 mm at 18–24/16–32 weeks, for PTB <32 weeks better prediction [103, 123]. The South Korea study showed that one could differentiate cerclage needs to avoid delivery <32 weeks by pretreatment elastography IO, and 1 week post-P_4 treatment EO assessment, showing significantly higher area under curve (AUC) than CL alone (0.858; P = 0.041), with sPTB delay/avoidance. P_4 direct contact with cervical matrix structures explains the better effects on EO at 1 week post-P_4 treatment, and women with no improvement in IO and EO after 1 week, possibly undergo progressive cervical softening.

5.2 Cervical cerclage, cervical pessary for preterm birth prevention

The mechanical support for an incompetent cervix has a long history, Cochrane Database of Systematic Reviews [124] presents three decisions for cervical cerclage, based on late miscarriages/sPTB history, short cervix ≤25 mm or open/dilated, with bulging membranes risking PROM, at ordinary ultrasound. Cerclage reduces sPTB risk by about 30% in women with a history of sPTB and short cervix, although at least one in three of these women still delivers preterm, as meta-analysis on individual patient-level data shows [125]. Cochrane Database of Systematic Reviews [126] showed that cerclage vs. no cerclage reduced the number of birth <37, <34 weeks (average RR: 0.77, 95% CI: 0.66–0.89) and <28 completed weeks gestation; and probably perinatal death risks.

Stiffness assessment favors a test for cerclage decision by "missing effect of vaginal P_4 on cervical stroma remodeling", and continuous cervical softness and shortness (even when CL < 10 mm) with sPTB high risks. A USA multicenter study revealed a gestational age at delivery significantly increased after 34 weeks, when CL < 10 mm while on P_4 and cerclage vs. without cerclage, but on vaginal P_4 (34^{+3days} weeks vs. 27^{+2days} weeks; P < 0.001), and lower rate sPTB at <37, 35, 32, 28, and 24 weeks in cerclage group (44.1 vs. 84.2%; 38.2 vs. 81.6%; 23.5 vs. 78.9%; 14.7 vs. 63.2%, and 11.8 vs. 39.5%; better neonatal outcomes parallel recorded) [127]. Cerclage decreases local levels of proinflammatory cytokines, adjuvant to P_4, and offers a biochemical barrier to membranes, effects added to mechanical support [128]. Post-cerclage CL assessment is very important, according to PTB high risk after elective cerclage vs. general population [129], and a CL ≤ 25 mm after cerclage can make the prognosis differences for the delivery before or after 32 weeks: 91.0% sensitivity, and 30.0% specificity [130], shortening progresses on softness, imposing P_4 continuation postcerclage, and a second/"reinforcing" cerclage to delay delivery [131], being mentioned also when amniotic membrane prolapse to or past the level of initial cerclage placement (visualized by direct speculum/ultrasound) [132]. Second/reinforcement stitch placement is an attempt to prolong pregnancy, imposing much caution, for maternal safety, and to avoid fetal inflammatory syndrome risks [133]. FIGO recommends stitch removal at 36–37 weeks [134] when everything is under medical control.

Vaginal microecology and immunity have great importance for cerclage outcomes [135], the epithelium protective effects on cervical stroma premature progression to ripening is not sufficient when abnormal vaginal microbiota, being recommended vaginal probiotics/eubiotics, according to *Lactobacillus acidophilus* known protective effects [136], topic therapy against bacterial vaginosis.

Cervical pessaries have a long history since 1961 [137], being reloaded according to new materials and technologies. A meta-analysis for PTB prevention <34 weeks vs. controls revealed that pessary shows a lack in prevention efficacy [138], without the possibility of determining inferiority, when compared to other methods because of studies heterogeneity. When short cervix (<25 mm), P_4 works as cerclage [124], confirmed by meta-analyses on singleton [139], and twins, with sPTB history [140], and better than pessary [141], that sustains utero-cervical angle [20]. P_4 was added to pessary when a shorter cervix (below 10th percentile) than in a previous sPTB (below 3rd percentile) was not more efficient, did not reduce birth rate <28, <32, <34, or <37 weeks gestation compared with pessary alone, in a German cohort study [142]. The Canadian Soc. Obstet. Gynecol. (2020) Guideline No. 398 [143] specifies that in women with a short cervix (<25 mm), when P_4 is used for PTB prevention, additional therapies as cervical cerclage (with the exception of a rescue cerclage for an examination-based diagnosis) or a pessary are not recommended (strong/moderate). The choice of treatment in Canada depends on adverse events, interventions cost-effectiveness, and patient/physician's preferences.

RCT systematic review from Cochrane Pregnancy and Childbirth's Trials Register, Clinical Trials.gov and WHO International Clinical Trials Registry Platform to 22 September 2021, evaluated pessaries benefits and harms in preventing sPTB (<34, 37 weeks gestation) compared to no treatment, vaginal P_4, cervical cerclage or bed-rest [144] revealed that pessary may reduce sPTB risks vs. no treatment [<34 weeks (RR: 0.72, 95% CI: 0.33–1.55); <37 weeks (RR: 0.68, 95% CI: 0.44–1.05), with low-certainty evidence for studies]; or vs. P_4 [<34 weeks (RR: 0.72, 95% CI 0.52–1.02); <37 weeks (RR: 0.89, 95% CI 0.73–1.09), with moderate certainty evidence for studies]; has little or no effect on maternal infection/inflammation risks (RR: 1.04, 95% CI 0.87–1.26); the comparison to cerclage was unclear, from o single study.

5.3 Progesterone, cerclage, pessary for reducing preterm birth risk

Perinatal outcomes of all three therapeutic opportunities are compared by a multination study [145], on three patient cohorts treated with cerclage (142, USA), vaginal P_4 (59, UK), and pessary (42, Spain). The results showed no statistic significant difference in perinatal loss, neonatal morbidity, and sPTB among the three groups, apart from a higher rate of sPTB < 34 weeks, after vaginal P_4 treatment in comparison to pessary (32% vs. 12%; RR: 2.70; 95% CI: 1.10–6.67). When one compared only subgroups with CL < 25 mm, irrespective GA, the difference between these two cohorts was not statistically significant (RR: 2.21; 95% CI: 0.83–5.89).

In sPTB < 34 weeks, the three procedures are recommended mainly when cervical softness is not accurately known, when vaginal P_4 fails, when CL after cerclage is below 15/10 mm, and one tries pregnancy prolongation by pessary adding, fetal high prematurity avoidance, without maternal and/or fetal risks. A Romanian retrospective study [65] compared PTB reduction, neonatal and maternal outcomes when short cervix (11–25 mm, and <10 mm at $14\text{–}23^{+6}$ weeks), in cases treated with vaginal P_4 and cerclage (8 patients, no CL < 10 mm), vaginal P_4 and pessary (62 cases, 10 with CL < 10 mm), and vaginal P_4, cerclage, and pessary (13 cases, 3 with CL < 10 mm). P_4 was administered from 6 weeks gestation, 200 mg/day, up to 36^{+6} weeks, bedtime, with supplementation at 16 weeks, or when was considered necessary, pessary was added when postcerclage CL was ≤25 mm. It was recorded pregnancy prolongation >34 weeks ($P < 0.0001$) when early administered vaginal P_4, and P_4 increased cerclage or/and of pessary benefits, better neonatal outcome (fetal weight, Apgar score ≥ 7, $P < 0.05$), reduced neonatal morbidity (only RDS, $P < 0.05$). All three methods were applied in sPTB before 34 weeks very high risks; average gestational age at delivery was 34.91 weeks vs. 37.37 weeks—P_4 and cerclage; 36.58 weeks: P_4 and pessary, when late administration of vaginal P_4, or when P_4 did not influence cervical remodeling. A retrospective cohort multicenter study [146] compared three therapeutic opportunities in four groups of pregnancies, at 15–29 weeks gestation, with CL ≤ 25 mm: A—P_4 vaginal, cerclage, pessary ([18], with highest risk for sPTB, and shortest cervix; median (range) 14.5 (0–25)); B—P_4 vaginal, and pessary ([141], CL: median (range) 15 (0–25)]); C—P_4 vaginal, and cerclage ([38], CL: median: 15.5 (0–25)); D—P_4 vaginal ([110], CL: median: 19 (2–25)). The rate of sPTB < 37 weeks was similar: 44.4% vs. 32.5% vs. 36.8% vs. 32.7% ($P = 0.665$). Their conclusion was that a combined rescue therapy involving vaginal P_4, cerclage, and pessary emerges as a promising management strategy when a short cervix and background history for sPTB high risk; pregnancy prolongation was safe.

5.4 New proposals for premature cervical remodeling prevention

There is still much work to understand how well therapy may better influence cervix consistency at cellular and microscopic level, what drug/material can restore stiffness, and sustain IO, ECM, and CSMCs/sphincter on increasing stress/stretch up to 37^{+1day} weeks. There were proposed/tested biomaterials, biodegradable and biocompatible for intracervical injection in rats—purified silk protein-polyethylene glycol, for intrinsic cervix reinforcement/augmentation with no other interference on structure, and to permit labor dilation, not extrinsic as pessary or cerclage [147], or to propose adult stem cells with their bioactive molecules to reinforce cervix, IO sphincter, as intraurethral/intrasphincterian use for postpartum stress urinary incontinence.

6. Conclusions for everyday practice

Gestational CR is difficult to accurately predict for individual cases. Usage of serial ultrasound (16–23^{+6} weeks) for CL, resistant CL when funneling, cervical mucus plug distance, and cervical sliding sign are beneficial, when new techniques for cervical stiffness assessment (such as ultrasound strain elastography, SWEI) are not available for sPTB risk accurate prediction, or for vaginal progesterone failure in short cervix syndrome. Softness may be an alert sign for fetus abnormalities, membranes, and amniotic fluid, not only per se. Vaginal microbiota evaluation and correction for Döderlein bacilli presence is very important, associated with vaginal progesterone, with positive effects on vaginal and cervical inflammations reduction. Actually, vaginal micronized progesterone is a strong recommendation for short cervix <25 mm, in asymptomatic cases, for history of recurrent late pregnancy loss, sPTB <34, and < 37 weeks, with singleton/twins, being proved no adverse effect on offspring, cerclage (one/two stitches) and pessary are second or third line option, with CL, and stiffness monitoring after procedure, without stopping progesterone up to 36^{+6} weeks, to avoid prematurity, if mother's health permits; all three therapies may be used when high risks for sPTB, with advanced cervical changes, even when CL < 10 mm.

Author details

Manuela Cristina Russu*, Adriana Elena Ghelmene, Ruxandra Viorica Stănculescu and Şerban Nastasia
"Carol Davila" University of Medicine and Pharmacy, Bucharest, Romania

*Address all correspondence to: manuela_russu@yahoo.com

References

[1] O' Brien MC, Vargis E, Paria CB, Reese J, et al. Raman spectroscopy provides a non-invasive approach for determining biochemical composition of the pregnant cervix *in vivo*. Acta Paediatrica. 2014;**102**(7):715-721

[2] Romero R, Dey SK, Fisher SJ. Preterm labor: One syndrome, many causes. Science. 2014;**345**(6198):760-765. DOI: 10.1126/science.1251816

[3] Smith R. Parturition. The New England Journal of Medicine. 2007;**356**:271-283

[4] Vink J, Feltovich H. Cervical etiology of spontaneous preterm birth. Seminars in Fetal and Neonatal Medicine. 2016;**21**(2):106-112. DOI: 10.1016/j.siny.2015.12.009

[5] Barros FC, Papageorghiou AT, Victora CG, Noble JA, Kramer MS, et al. The distribution of clinical phenotypes of preterm birth syndrome: Implications for prevention. JAMA Pediatrics. 2015;**169**:220-229

[6] Chawanpaiboon S, Vogel J, et al. Global, regional, and national estimates of levels of preterm birth in 2014: A systematic review and modelling analysis. Lancet Global Health. 2019;7:e37-e46. DOI: 10.1016/S2214-109X(18)30451-0

[7] Mangham JL, Petrou S, Doyle WL, Draper SE, Marlow N. The cost of preterm birth throughout childhood in England and Wales. Pediatrics. Feb 2009;**123**(2):e312-e327

[8] Cabrera-Garcia L, Cruz-Melqquizo S, Ruiz-Antorán B, Torres F, Avendaño-Solã C, et al. PESAPRO trial group. Evaluation of two treatment strategies for the prevention of preterm birth in women identified as at risk by ultrasound (PESAPRO trial): Study protocol for a randomized controlled trial. Trials. 2015;**16**:427. DOI: 10.1186/s13063-015-0964-y

[9] Read CP, Word RA, Ruscheinsky MA, Timmons BC, Mahendroo M. Cervical remodeling during pregnancy and parturition: Molecular characterization of the softening phase in mice. Reproduction. 2007;**134**(2):327-340

[10] Myers KM, Feltovich H, Mazza E, Vink J, House M, et al. The mechanical role of the cervix in pregnancy. Journal of Biomechanics. 2015;**48**:1511-1523. DOI: 10.1016/j.jbiomech.2015.02.065

[11] American College of Obstetricians and Gynecologists. Practice bulletin No. 142: Cerclage for the management of cervical insufficiency. Obstetrics & Gynecology. 2014;**123**(2Pt1):372-379

[12] Danforth D. The fibrous nature of the human cervix and its relation to the isthmic segment in gravid and nongravid uteri. The Proceedings of the Institute of Medicine of Chicago. 1947;**16**(10):295

[13] Iams JD. Clinical practice. Prevention of preterm parturition. The New England Journal of Medicine. 2014;**370**:254-261

[14] Yao W, Gan KM, Myers KM, Vink JY, Hendon CP, et al. Collagen fiber orientation and dispersion in the upper cervix of non-pregnant and pregnant women. PLoS One. 2016;**11**(11):e0166709. DOI: 10.1371/journal.pone.0166709

[15] Timmons B, Akins M, Mahendroo M. Cervical remodeling during pregnancy and parturition. Trends in Endocrinology

and Metabolism. 2010;**21**(6):353-361. DOI: 10.1016/1.tem.2010.01.011

[16] Lau TY, Sangha HK, Chien EK, Mcfarlin BL, Toussaint KC, et al. Application of Fourier transform-second-harmonic generation imaging to the rat cervix. Journal of Microscopy. 2013;**251**:77-83. DOI: 10.1111/jmi.12046

[17] Bank RA, Tekoppele JM, Janus GJ, Wassen MH, Sakkers RJ, et al. Pyridinium cross-links in bone of patients with osteogenesis imperfecta: Evidence of a normal intrafibrillar collagen packing. Journal of Bone and Mineral Research. 2000;**15**:1330-1336

[18] Aspden RM. Collagen organization in the cervix and its relation to mechanical function. Collagen and Related Research. 1988;**8**:103-112

[19] Vink J, Myers KM. Cervical alterations in pregnancy. Best Practice & Research Clinical Obstetrics & Gynaecology. Oct 2018;**52**:88-102. DOI: 10.1016/j.bpobgyn.2018.03.007

[20] House M, Kaplan D, Socrate S. Relationships between mechanical properties and extracellular matrix constituents of the cervical stroma during pregnancy. Seminars in Perinatology. 2009;**33**:300-307

[21] Myers K, Socrate S, Tzeranis D, House M. Changes in the biochemical constituents and morphologic appearance of the human cervical stroma during pregnancy. European Journal of Obstetrics, Gynecology, and Reproductive Biology. 2009;**144**(Suppl. 1):S82-S89

[22] Zork NM, Myers KM, Yoshida K, et al. A systematic evaluation of collagen cross-links in the human cervix. American Journal of Obstetrics and Gynecology. 2015;**212**(321):e1-e8

[23] Fernandez M, House M, Jambawalikar S, et al. Investigating the mechanical function of the cervix during pregnancy using finite element models derived from high-resolution 3D MRI. Computer Methods in Biomechanics and Biomedical Engineering. 2016;**19**(4):404-417. DOI: 10.1080/10255842.2015.1033163

[24] Nallasamy S, Yoshida K, Akins M, Myers K, Mahendroo M, et al. Steroid hormones are key modulators of tissue mechanical function via regulation of collagen and elastic fibers. Endocrinology. 2017;**158**:950-962. DOI: 10.1210/en.2016-1930

[25] Yoshida K, Jayyosi C, Lee N, Mahendroo M, Myers KM. Mechanics of cervical remodeling: Insights from rodent models of pregnancy. Interface Focus. 2019;**9**(5):20190026. DOI: 10.1098/rsfs.2019.0026

[26] Svensson L, Narlid I, Oldberg A. Fibromodulin and lumican bind to the same region on collagen type I fibrils. FEBS Letters. 2000;**470**:178-182

[27] Danforth DN. The distribution and functional activity of the cervical musculature. American Journal of Obstetrics and Gynecology. 1954;**68**:1261-1271

[28] Pajntar M. The smooth muscles of the cervix in labour. European Journal of Obstetrics, Gynecology, and Reproductive Biology. 1994;**55**:9-12. DOI: 10.1016/0028-2243(94)90180-5

[29] Leppert PC. Anatomy and physiology of cervical ripening. Clinical Obstetrics and Gynecology. 1995;**38**(2):267-279

[30] Vink JY, Quin S, Brock CO, Kitajewski JK, Gallos G, et al. A new paradigm for the role of smooth muscle cells in the human cervix. Obstetrics.

2016;**215**(4):478.e1-478.e11. DOI: 10.1016/j.ajog.2016.04.053

[31] Pajntar M, Leskosek B, Rudel D, Verdenik I. Contribution of cervical smooth muscle activity to the duration of latent and active phases of labor. British Journal of Obstetrics and Gynaecology. 2001;**108**:533-538

[32] Ferland DJ, Darios ES, Watts SW. The persistence of active smooth muscle in the female rat cervix through pregnancy. American Journal of Obstetrics and Gynecology. 2015;**212**(2):244.e1-244.e8

[33] Timmons BC, Mahendroo M. Timing of neutrophil activation and expression of proinflammatory markers do not support a role for neutrophils in cervical ripening in the mouse. Biology of Reproduction. 2006;**74**:236-245

[34] Hunter PJ, Sheikh S, David AL, Peebles DM, Klein N. Cervical leukocytes and spontaneous preterm birth. Journal of Reproductive Immunology. 2016;**113**:42-49

[35] Yellon SM, Dobyns AE, Beck HL, Kurtzman JT, Kirby MA, et al. Loss of progesterone receptor-mediated actions induce preterm cellular and structural remodeling of the cervix and premature birth. PLoS One. 2018;**8**(12):e81340. DOI: 10.1371/journal.pone.0081340. eCollection2013

[36] Akins ML, Luby-Phelps K, Bank RA, Mahendroo M. Cervical softening during pregnancy: Regulated changes in collagen cross-linking and composition of matricellular proteins in the mouse. Biology of Reproduction. 2011;**84**:1053-1062

[37] Mahendroo M. Cervical remodeling in term and preterm birth: Insights from an animal model. Reproduction. 2012;**143**(4):429-438

[38] Shi L, Hu L, Lee N, Fang S, Myers K. Three dimensional anisotropic hyperelastic constitutive model describing the mechanical response of human and mouse model. Acta Biomaterialia. 2022;**150**:277-294. DOI: 10.1016/j.actbio.2022.07.062

[39] Word RA, Li X-H, Hnat M, Carrick K. Dynamics of cervical remodeling during pregnancy and parturition: Mechanisms and current concepts. Seminars in Reproductive Medicine. 2007;**25**:69-79

[40] Torres J, Faris I, Callejas A. Histobiomechanical remodeling of the cervix during pregnancy: Proposed framework. Mathematical Problems in Engineering. 2019;**2019**. Article ID: 5957432. DOI: 10.1155/2019/5957432

[41] Humphrey JD, Rajagopal KR. A constrained mixture model for growth and remodeling of soft tissues. Mathematical Models and Methods in Applied Sciences. 2002;**12**:407-430. DOI: 10.1142/S0218202502001714

[42] Humphrey JD. Constrained mixture models of soft tissue growth and remodeling. Twenty years after. Journal of Elasticity. 2021;**145**(1-2):49-75. DOI: 10.1007/s10659-020-09809

[43] Holt R, Timmons BC, Akgul Y, Akins ML, Mahendroo M. The molecular mechanisms of cervical ripening differ between term and preterm birth. Endocrinology. 2011;**152**(3):1036-1046

[44] Hassan S, Romero R, Tarca AL, Nhan-Chang CL, Kim CJ, et al. The transcriptome of cervical ripening in human pregnancy before the onset of labor at term: Identification of novel molecular functions involved in this process. Journal

of Maternal-Fetal & Neonatal Medicine. 2009;**22**:1183-1193

[45] Elovitz MA, Brown AG, Anton L, Gilstrop M, Bastek J, et al. Distinct cervical microRNA profiles are present in women destined to have a preterm birth. American Journal of Obstetrics and Gynecology. 2014;**210**(221):e1-e11

[46] Feltovich H, Hall TJ, Berghella V. Beyond cervical length: Emerging technologies for assessing the pregnant cervix. American Journal of Obstetrics and Gynecology. 2012;**207**(5):345-354

[47] Winkler M, Rath W. Changes in extracellular matrix during pregnancy and parturition. Journal of Perinatal Medicine. 1999;**27**(1):45-61. DOI: 20.1515/JPN.1999.006

[48] Gonzalez JM, Xu H, Chai J, Ofori E, Elovitz MA. Preterm and term cervical ripening in CD1 mice (*Mus musculus*): Similar or divergent molecular mechanisms? Biology of Reproduction. 2009;**81**:1226-1232

[49] Rath W, Osmers R, Adelmann-Grill BC, Szeverini M, et al. Principles of physiologic and drug-induced cervix ripening--recent morphologic and biochemical findings. Geburtshilfe und Frauenheilkunde. 1990;**50**(9):657-664

[50] Jorge S, Chang S, Barzilai JJ, Leppert P, Segars JH. Mechanical signaling in reproductive tissues: Mechanisms and importance. Reproductive Sciences. 2014;**21**(9):1093-1107

[51] Myers KM, Paskaleva AP, House M, Socrate S. Mechanical and biochemical properties of human cervical tissue. Acta Biomaterialia. 2008;**4**(1):104-116

[52] Buhimschi IA, Dussably L, Buhimschi CS, Ahmed A, Weiner CP. Physical and biomechanical characteristics of rat cervical ripening are not consistent with increased collagenase activity. American Journal of Obstetrics and Gynecology. 2004;**19**:1695-1704

[53] Badir S, Mazza E, Zimmermann R, Bajka M. Cervical softening occurs early in pregnancy: Characterization of cervical stiffness in 100 healthy women using the aspiration technique. Prenatal Diagnosis. 2013;**33**:737-741. DOI: 10.1002/pd. 4116

[54] Iams JD, Goldenberg RL, Meis PJ, Mercer BM, Roberts JM, et al. The length of the cervix and the risk of spontaneous premature delivery. National Institute of Child Health and Human Development maternal Fetal medicine unit network. The New England Journal of Medicine. 1996;**334**:567-572

[55] Bortoletto TG, Silva TV, Borovac-Pinheiro A, Pereira CM, Pacagnella RC, et al. Cervical length varies considering different populations and gestational outcomes. Results from a systematic review and meta-analysis. PLoS One. 2021;**16**(2):e0245746. DOI: 10.1371/journal.pone.0245746. eCollection2021

[56] House M, Socrate S. The cervix as a biomechanical structure. Ultrasound in Obstetrics & Gynecology. 2006;**28**:745-749

[57] Zilianti M, Azuaga A, Calderon F, Mendoza G, et al. Monitoring the effacement of the uterine cervix by transperineal sonography: A new perspective. Journal of Ultrasound in Medicine. 1995;**14**:719-724

[58] Fernandez M, Vink J, Yoshida K, Wapner R, Myers K. Direct measurement of the permeability of human cervical

tissue. Journal of Biomechanical Engineering. 2013;**135**:021024

[59] Tantengco OAG, Menon R. Contractile function of the cervix plays a role in normal and pathological pregnancy and parturition. Medical Hypotheses. 2020;**145**:110336. DOI: 10.1016/j.mehy.2020.110336

[60] Leppert PC. Proliferation and apoptosis of fibroblasts and smooth muscle cells in rat uterine cervix throughout gestation and the effect of the antiprogesterone onapristone. American Journal of Obstetrics and Gynecology. 1998;**178**(7):13-25

[61] Vink J, Qin S, Praditpan P, Ananth CV, Myers K, et al. Human cervical smooth muscle stretch increases matrix metalloproteinase secretion: A new mechanism to explain premature cervical remodeling. American Journal of Obstetrics and Gynecology. 2016;**214**:S122. DOI: 10.1016/j.ajog.2015.10.238

[62] Mourad M, Qin S, Ananth CV, Fu A, Myers K, et al. Human cervical smooth muscle stretch increases pro-inflammatory cytokine secretion. American Journal of Obstetrics and Gynecology. 2017;**216**:S77-S78. DOI: 10.1016/j.ajog.2016.11.999

[63] Vink J, Yu V, Dahal S, Lohner J, Gallos G, et al. Extracellular matrix rigidity modulates human cervical smooth muscle contractility. New insights into premature cervical failire and spontaneous preterm birth. Reproductive Sciences. 2021;**28**(1):237-251. DOI: 10.1007/s43032-020-00268-6

[64] Mancuso MS, Szychowski JM, Owen J, et al. Vaginal ultrasound trial consortium. Cervical funneling: Effect on gestational length and ultrasound-indicated cerclage in high-risk women. American Journal of Obstetrics and Gynecology. 2010;**203**(259):e1-e5

[65] Russu M, Ghelmene A, Nastasia Ş. Vaginal progesterone, cerclage, pessary for premature cervical remodeling and preterm birth prevention; Pregnancy outcome. In: Oral Presentation at Virtual 19th World Congress of Gynecological Endocrinology, Florence, Italy. International Society of Endocrinological Gynecology (ISGE), Biomedical Technologies SRL; 3-5 Dec 2020. Available from: https://isge2020.isgesociety.com/scientific-program/

[66] Tsikouras P, Anastasopoulos G, Maroulis V, Bothou A, Teichmann AT, et al. Comparative evaluation of Arabin pessary and cervical cerclage for the prevention of preterm labor in asymptomatic women with high risk factors. International Journal of Environmental Research and Public Health. 2016;**15**(4):791. DOI: 10.3390/jepbh15040791

[67] Kusanovic JP, Espinoza J, Romero R, Gonçalves LF, Hassan SS, et al. Clinical significance of the presence of amniotic fluid 'sludge' in asymptomatic patients at high risk for spontaneous preterm delivery. Ultrasound in Obstetrics & Gynecology. 2007;**30**(5):706-714

[68] Elovitz MA, Wang Z, Chien EK, Rychllik DF, Phillippe M. A new model inflammation-induced preterm birth: The role of platelet activated factor and toll-like receptor-4. American Journal of Pathology. 2003;**163**:2103-2111

[69] Maradny EE, Kanayama N, Halim A, Maehara K, Terao T. Effects of neutrophil chemotactic factors on cervical ripening. Clinical and Experimental Obstetrics & Gynecology. 1995;**22**:76-85

[70] Yellon MS. Contribution to the dynamics of cervix remodeling prior

to term and preterm birth. Biology of Reproduction. 2017;**96**(1):13-23. DOI: 10.1095/biolreprod.116.142844

[71] Nallasamy S, Akins M, Tetreault B, Luby-Phelps K, Mahendroo M. Distinct reorganization of collagen architecture in lipopolysaccharide-mediated premature cervical remodeling. Biology of Reproduction. 2018;**98**:63-74. DOI: 10.1093/biolre/iox155

[72] Yellon MS. Immunobiology of cervix ripening. Frontiers in Immunology. 2020;**10**:3156. DOI: 10.3389/fimmu.2019.03156.eCollection2019

[73] Timmons BC, Fairhurst AM, Mahendroo MS. Temporal changes in myeloid cells in the cervix during pregnancy and parturition. Journal of Immunology. 2009;**182**(5):2700-2707. DOI: 10.4049/jimmunol.0803138

[74] Payne JK, Clyde AL, Weldon JA, Milford T-A, Yellon MS. Residency and activation of myeloid cells during remodeling of the prepartum murine cervix. Biology of Reproduction. 2012;**87**:106

[75] Törnblom SA, Klimaviciute A, Bystrom B, Chromek M, Ekman-Ordeberg G, et al. Non-infected preterm parturition is related to increased concentrations of IL-6, IL-8 and MCP-1 in human cervix. Reproductive Biology and Endocrinology. 2005;**3**:39. DOI: 10.1186/1477-7827-3-39

[76] Timmons BC, Reese J, Socrate S, Ehinger N, Mahendroo M, et al. Prostaglandins are essential for cervical ripening in LPS-mediated preterm birth but not term or antiprogestin-driven preterm ripening. Endocrinology. 2014;**155**:287-298

[77] Gudicha DW, Romero R, Gomez-Lopez N, Galaz J, Tarca A, et al. The amniotic fluid proteome predicts imminent preterm delivery in asymptomatic women with a short cervix. Scientific Reports. 2022;**12**(1):11781. DOI: 10.1038/s41598-022-15392-3

[78] Cullen BM, Harkness RD. The effect of hormones on the physical properties and collagen content of the rat's uterine cervix. The Journal of Physiology. 1960;**152**:419-436. DOI: 10.1113/jphysiol.1960.sp006497

[79] Vink J, Dahal S, Li H, Sheetz M, Wapner R, Gallos G. Progesterone decreases human cervical smooth muscle cell (HCSMC) contractility. American Journal of Obstetrics and Gynecology. 2019;**220**(Suppl. 1):S372. DOI: 10.1015/j.ajog.2018.11.579

[80] Tripathy S, Nallasamy S, Mahendroo M. Progesterone and its receptor signaling in cervical remodeling: Mechanisms of physiological actions and therapeutic implications. Journal of Steroid Biochemistry and Molecular Biology. 2022;**223**:106137. DOI: 10.1016/j.jsbmb.2022.106137

[81] House M, Tadesse-Telila S, Norwitz ER, Socrate S, Kaplan DL. Inhibitory effect of progesterone on cervical tissue formation in a three-dimensional culture system with human cervical fibroblasts. Biology of Reproduction. 2014;**90**(1):18

[82] Carbonne B, Dallot E, Haddad B, Ferré F, Cabrol D. Effects of progesterone on prostaglandin E(2)-induced changes in glycosaminoglycan synthesis by human cervical fibroblasts in culture. Molecular Human Reproduction. 2000;**6**(7):661-664

[83] Nold C, Maubert M, Anton L, Yellon S, Elovitz MA. Prevention of

preterm birth by progestational agents: What are the molecular mechanisms? American Journal of Obstetrics and Gynecology. 2013;**208**(3):223.e1-223.e7

[84] Kirby MA, Heuerman AC, Custer M, Dobyns AE, Yellon SM, et al. Progesterone receptor-mediated actions regulate remodeling of the cervix in preparation for preterm parturition. Reproductive Sciences. 2016;**23**(11):1473-1483. DOI: 10.1177/1933719116650756

[85] Heuerman AC, Hollinger TT, Menon R, Mesiano S, Yellon SM. Cervix stromal cells and the progesterone receptor a isoform mediate effects of progesterone for prepartum Remodeling. Reproductive Sciences. 2019;**26**(5):690-696. DOI: 10.1177/1933719118820462

[86] Sugita Y, Kuwabara Y, Katayama A, Matsuda S, Oishi Y, et al. Characteristic impairment of progesterone response in cultured cervical fibroblasts obtained from patients with refractory cervical insufficiency. Scientific Reports. 2023;**13**(1):11709. DOI: 10.1038/s41598-023-37732-7

[87] Bishop EH. Pelvic scoring for elective induction. Obstetrics and Gynecology. 1964;**24**:266-268

[88] Yan Y, Gomez-Loez N, Hernandez-Andrade E, Hassan SS, Romero R, et al. Photoacoustic imaging of the uterine cervix to assess collagen and water content changes in murine pregnancy. Biomedical Optics Express. 2019;**10**(9):4643-4655. DOI: 10.1364/BOE.10.004643

[89] Hassan SS, Romero R, Berry SM, Dang K, Wolfe HM, et al. Patients with an ultrasonographic cervical length 15 mm have nearly a 50% risk of early spontaneous preterm delivery. American Journal of Obstetrics and Gynecology. 2000;**182**:1458-1467. DOI: 10.1067/mob.2000.106851

[90] Volpe N, Schera GBL, Dall'Astra A, Frusca T, et al. Cervical sliding sign: New sonographyc marker to predict impeding preterm delivery in women with uterine contractions. Ultrasound in Obstetrics & Gynecology. 2019;**54**(4):557-558. DOI: 10.1002/nog.2039524.23

[91] Becher N, Waldorf KA, Hein M, Uldbjerg N. The cervical mucus plug: Structured review of the literature. Acta Obstetricia et Gynecologica Scandinavica. 2009;**88**:502-513

[92] Vaisbuch E, Romero R, Erez O, Kusanovic JP, Hassan SS, et al. Clinical significance of early (<20 weeks) vs. late (20-24 weeks) detection of sonographic short cervix in asymptomatic women in the mid-trimester. Ultrasound in Obstetrics & Gynecology. 2010;**36**(4):471-481

[93] Miller ES, Tita AT, Grobman WA. Second-trimester cervical length screening among asymptomatic women: An evaluation of risk-based strategies. Obstetrics and Gynecology. 2015;**126**:61-66

[94] Berghella V, Saccone G, Cochrane Pregnancy and Childbirth Group. Cervical assessment by ultrasound for preventing preterm delivery. Cochrane Database of Systematic Reviews. 2019;**9**(9):CD007235. DOI: 10.1002/14651858

[95] Feltovich H, Nam K, Hall TJ. Quantitative ultrasound assessment of cervical microstructure. Ultrasound imaging. 2010;**32**(3):131-142. DOI: 10.1177/016173461003200302

[96] Nejim Z, Navaro L, Morin C. Badel P quantitative analysis of second harmonic generated images of collagen fibers; a review. Research on Biomedical Engineering. 2023;**39**:273-293

[97] Clark-Patterson G, Domingo M, Miller SK. Biomechanics of pregnancy and vaginal delivery. Current Opinion in Biomedical Engineering. 2022;**22**:100386

[98] Hernandez-Andrade E, Romero R, Korzeniewski SJ, Hassan S, et al. Cervical strain determined by ultrasound elastography and its association with spontaneous preterm delivery. Journal of Perinatal Medicine. 2014;**42**(2):159-169. DOI: 10/1515/jpm-2013-0277

[99] Hee L, Liao D, Sandager P, Gregersen H, Uldbjerg N. Cervical stiffness evaluated in vivo by endoflip in pregnant women. PLoS One. 2014;**9**:e91121

[100] Hernandez-Andrade E, Hassan SS, Ahn H, Korzeniewski SJ, Chaiworapongsa T, et al. Evaluation of cervical stiffness during pregnancy using semiquantitative ultrasound elastography. Ultrasound in Obstetrics & Gynecology. 2013;**41**:152-161

[101] Feltovich H, Carlson L. New techniques in evaluation of the cervix. Seminars in Perinatology. 2017;**41**(8):4 77-484. DOI: 10.1053/j. semperi.2017.08.006

[102] O'Hara S, Zelesco M, Sun Z. Shear wave elastography of the maternal cervix. Journal of Ultrasound in Medicine. 2021;**40**(4):701-714

[103] Hernandez-Andrade E, Maymon E, Luewan S, Hassan SS, Romero R, et al. A soft cervix, categorized by shear-wave elastography, in women with short or with normal cervical length at 18-24 weeks is associated with a higher prevalence of spontaneous preterm delivery. Journal of Perinatal Medicine. 2018;**46**(5):489-501. DOI: 10.1515/ jpm-2018-0062

[104] Muller M, Aït-Belkacem D, Hessabi M, Gennisson JL, Tsatsaris V, et al. Assessment of the cervix in pregnant women using shear wave elastography: A feasibility study. Ultrasound in Medicine & Biology. 2015;**41**(11):2789-2797

[105] Carlson LC, Hall TJ, Rosado-Mendez IM, Mao L, Feltovich H. Quantitative assessment of cervical softening during pregnancy with shear wave elasticity imaging: An *in vivo* longitudinal study. Interface Focus. 2019;**9**(5):20190030. DOI: 10.1098/ rsfs.2019.0030

[106] Hernandez-Andrade E, Aurioles-Garibay A, Chaiworapongsa T, Hassan SS, Romero R, et al. Effect of depth on shear-wave elastography estimated in the internal and external cervical os during pregnancy. Journal of Perinatal Medicine. 2014;**42**(5):549-557

[107] Carlson LC, Hall TJ, Rosado-Mendez LM, Feltovich H, et al. Detection of changes in cervical softness using shear wave speed in early versus late pregnancy: An in vivo cross-sectional study. Ultrasound in Medicine & Biology. 2018;**44**(3):515-521

[108] Peralta L, Molina FS, Melchor J, Gomez LF, Rus G, et al. Transient elastography to assess the cervical ripening during pregnancy: A preliminary study. Ultraschall in der Medizin. 2017;**38**:395-402. DOI: 10.1055/s-0035-1553325

[109] Reusch LM, Feltovich H, Carlson LC, Hall G, Eliceiri KW, et al. Non linear optical microscopy and ultrasound imaging of human cervical structure. Journal of Biomedical Optics. 2013;**18**:031110

[110] Westervelt AR, Myers KM. Computer modeling tools to understand the causes of preterm birth. Seminars in Perinatology. 2017;**41**(8):485-492. DOI: 10.1053/semperi.2017.08.007

[111] Csapo A. Progesterone block. The American Journal of Anatomy.

1956;**98**(2):273-279. DOI: 10.1002/aja.1000980206

[112] Hassan SS, Romero R, Vidyadhari D, Fusey S, Sambarey P, et al. Vaginal progesterone reduces the rate of preterm birth in women with a sonographic short cervix. A multicenter, randomized, double blind, placebo-controlled trial. Ultrasound in Obstetrics & Gynecology. 2011;**38**(1):18-31

[113] Romero R, Nicolaides KH, Conde-Agudelo A, O'Brien JM, Hassan SS, et al. Vaginal progesterone decreases preterm birth ≤ 34 weeks of gestation in women with a singleton pregnancy, and a short cervix: An updated meta-analysis including data from the OPPTIMUM study. Ultrasound in Obstetrics & Gynecology. 2016;**48**(3):308-317

[114] Romero R, Conde-Agudelo A, Da Fonseca E, Hassan SS, Nicolaides KH, et al. Vaginal progesterone for preventing preterm birth, and adverse perinatal outcomes in singleton gestation with a short cervix. A meta-analysis of individual patient data. American Journal of Obstetrics and Gynecology. 2018;**218**:161-180. DOI: 10.10164/j.ajog.2017.11.576

[115] Luxenbourg D, Porat S, Romero R, Raif Nesher D, Kabiri D, et al. The effectiveness of vaginal progesterone in reducing preterm birth in high-risk patients diagnosed with short cervical length after 24 weeks: A retrospective cohort study. Frontiers in Medicine. 2023;**10**:1130942. DOI: 10.3389/fmed.2023.1130942.eCollection 2023

[116] Society for Maternal–Fetal Medicine Publications Committee, with assistance of Vincenzo Berghella. Progesterone and preterm birth prevention: Translating clinical trials data into clinical practice. American Journal of Obstetrics and Gynecology. 2012;**206**:56-86

[117] Norman JE, Marlow N, Messow CM, Shennan A, Bennett PR, Thornton S, et al. Vaginal progesterone prophylaxis for preterm birth (the OPPTIMUM study): A multicentre, randomized, double-blind trial. Lancet. 2016;**387**(10033):2106-2116

[118] D'Antonio F, Berghella V, Di Mascio D, Saccone G, Khalil A, et al. Role of progesterone, cerclage and pessary in preventing preterm birth in twin pregnancies: A systematic review and network meta-analysis. European Journal of Obstetrics, Gynecology, and Reproductive Biology. 2021;**261**:166-177. DOI: 10.1016/j.ejogrb.2021.04.023

[119] Norman JE, Bennett P. Preterm birth prevention-time to PROGRESS beyond progesterone. PLoS Medicine. 2017;**14**:e1002391

[120] Furcron AE, Romero R, Plazyo O, Unkel R, Gomez-Lopez N, et al. Vaginal progesterone, but not 17alpha-hydroxyprogesterone caproate, has antiinflammatory effects at the murine maternal-fetal interface. American Journal of Obstetrics and Gynecology. 2015;**213**(6):846.e1-846.e19. DOI: 10.1016/j.ajog.2015.08.010

[121] Zierden H, Ortiz IJ, Delong K, Ensign L. Enhanced drug delivery to the reproductive tract using nanomedicine reveals therapeutic options for prevention of preterm birth. Science Translational Medicine. 13 Jan 2021;**13**(576):eabc6245. DOI: 10.1126/scitranamed.abc6245

[122] Saccone G, Khalifeh A, Elimian A, Gahrami E, Berghella V, et al. Vaginal progesterone vs intramuscular 17α-hydroxyprogesterone caproate for prevention of recurrent spontaneous preterm birth in singleton gestations: Systematic review and meta-analysis of randomized controlled trials.

Ultrasound in Obstetrics & Gynecology. 2017;**49**(3):315-321

[123] JiY J, Kwon K, Kwon J-Y. The feasibility of cervical elastography in predicting preterm delivery in singleton pregnancy with short cervix following progesterone treatment. International Journal of Environmental Research and Public Health. 2021;**18**(4):2026. DOI: 10.3390/ijerph18042026

[124] Alfirevic Z, Stampalija T, Jorgensen AL, et al. Cervical stitch (cerclage) for preventing preterm birth in singleton pregnancy. Cochrane Database of Systematic Reviews. 2012;**4**:CD008991. DOI: 10.1002/1465858

[125] Berghella V, Rafael T, Szychowski J, Rust OA, Owen J. Cerclage for short cervix on ultrasound in singleton gestations with prior preterm birth: Meta-analysis of trials using individual patient-level data. Obstetrics and Gynecology. 2011;**117**:663-671

[126] Alfirevic Z, Stampalija T, Medley N. Cervical stitch (cerclage) for preventing preterm birth in singleton pregnancy. Cochrane Database of Systematic Reviews. 2017;**6**(6):CD008991. DOI: 10.1002/14651858.CD008991.pub3

[127] Enakpene CA, DiGiovanni L, Jones TN, Marshalla M, Della Torre M, et al. Cervical cerclage for singleton pregnant patients on vaginal progesterone with progressive cervical shortening. American Journal of Obstetrics and Gynecology. 2018;**219**(4):397.e1-397.e10. DOI: 10.1016/j. ajog.2018.06.020

[128] Monsanto SP, Dahne S, Ono E, Pendeloski KPT, Tayade C, et al. Cervical cerclage placement decreases local levels of proinflammatory cytokines in patients with cervical insufficiency. American Journal of Obstetrics and Gynecology. 2017;**217**(4):455.e1-455.e8. DOI: 10.1016/j. ajog.2017.06.024

[129] Nelson L, Dola T, Tran T, Dola C, et al. Pregnancy outcomes following placement of elective, urgent and emergent cerclage. The Journal of Maternal-Fetal & Neonatal Medicine. 2009;**22**:269-273

[130] Song RK, Cha HH, Roh CR. Post-cerclage ultrasonographic cervical length can predict preterm delivery in elective cervical cerclage patients. Obstetrics & Gynecology Science. 2016;**59**(1):17-23

[131] Baxter JK, Airoldi J, Berghella V. Short cervical length after history-indicated cerclage; is a reinforcing cerclage beneficial? American Journal of Obstetrics and Gynecology. 2005;**193**(3):1204-1207

[132] Simcox R, Shennan A. Reinforcing cerclage in the prevention of preterm birth in women at high risk; a retrospective case-controlled study. Australian and New Zealand Journal of Obstetrics and Gynaecology. 2012;**52**:224-228

[133] Jung E, Romero R, Yeo L, Diaz-Primera R, Hsu CD, et al. The fetal inflammatory response syndrome: The origins of a concept, pathophysiology, diagnosis, and obstetrical implications. Seminars in Fetal and Neonatal Medicine. 2020;**25**(4):101146

[134] Shennan A, Story L, Jacobsson B, Grobman AW. The FIGO working group for preterm birth. FIGO good practice recommendations on cervical cerclage for prevention of preterm birth. International Journal of Gynecology & Obstetrics. 2021;**155**(1):19-22. DOI: 10.1002/ijgo.13835

[135] Cai S, Wu Y, Zeng L, Ding Y. Effects of vaginal microecology and immunity on the pregnancy outcome of cervical cerclage. BMC Women's Health. 2022;**22**(1):167. DOI: 10.1186/s12905-022-01751-9

[136] Flavian F, Hezelgrave NL, Kanno T, Prosdocim DK, Tribe RM, et al. Cervico-vaginal microbiota and metabolome predict preterm birth risk in an ethnically diverse cohort. JCI Insight. 2021;**6**(16):e149257. DOI: 10.1172/jci.insight.149257

[137] Vitsky M. Simple treatment of the incompetent cervical *os*. American Journal of Obstetrics and Gynecology. 1961;**81**:1194-1197

[138] Correa DT, Amorin EG, Tomazelli JAG, Correa MD Jr. Use of the pessary in the prevention of preterm delivery. Revista Brasileira de Ginecologia e Obstetrícia. 2019;**41**(1):53-58

[139] Conde Aquidelo A, Romero R, Nicolaides KH, et al. Vaginal progesterone is as effective as cervical cerclage to prevent preterm birth in women with a singleton gestation, previous spontaneous preterm birth, and a short cervix: Updated indirect comparison meta-analysis. American Journal of Obstetrics and Gynecology. 2018;**219**(1):10-25

[140] Romero R, Conde Aquidelo A, El-Refaie VV, Hassan SS, Nicolaides KH, et al. Vaginal progesterone decreases preterm birth and neonatal morbidity and mortality in women with a twin gestation and a short cervix: An updated meta-analysis of individual patient data. Ultrasound in Obstetrics & Gynecology. 2017;**49**(3):303-314

[141] Conde-Agudelo A, Romero R, Nicolaides KH. Cervical pessary to prevent preterm birth in asymptomatic high-risk women: A systematic review and meta-analysis. American Journal of Obstetrics and Gynecology. 2020;**223**(1):42-65. e2. DOI: 10.1016/j.ajog.2019.12.266

[142] Stricker N, Timmesfeld N, Kyvernitakis I, Goerges J, Arabin B. Vaginal progesterone combined with cervical pessary: A chance for pregnancies at risk for preterm birth? American Journal of Obstetrics and Gynecology. 2016;**214**(6):739.e1-739.e10. DOI: 10.1016/j.ajog.2015.12.007

[143] Jain V, McDonald DS, Mundle RW, Farine D. Progesterone for prevention of spontaneous preterm birth. Journal of Obstetrics and Gynaecology Canada. 2020;**42**(6):806-812. DOI: 10.1016/j.jog.2019.04.012

[144] Abdel-Aleem H, Shaaban OM, Abdel-Aleem MA, Aboelfadle MA. Cervical pessary for preventing preterm birth in singleton pregnancies. Cochrane Review is a Systematic Review. 2022;**12**(12):CD014508. DOI: 10.1002/14651858.CD014508

[145] Alfirevic Z, Owen J, Carreras Moratonas E, Sharp AN, Goya M, et al. Vaginal progesterone, cerclage or cervical pessary for preventing preterm birth in asymptomatic singleton pregnant women with a history of preterm birth and a sonographic short cervix. Ultrasound in Obstetrics & Gynecology. 2013;**41**(2):146-151

[146] Shor S, Zimmerman A, Maymon R, Kovo M, Melcer Y, et al. Combined therapy with vaginal progesterone, Arabin cervical pessary, and cervical cerclage to prevent preterm delivery in high risk women. Journal of Maternal-Fetal & Neonatal Medicine. 2021;**34**(13):2154-2158. DOI: 10.1080/14767058.2019.1659771

[147] Feltovich H, House M. Innovative methods of cervical assessment and potential for novel treatment. Clinical Obstetrics and Gynecology. 2014;**57**(3):531-536. DOI: 10.1097/GRF.0000000000000049

Section 2

Labor Outcome

Chapter 3

Second Stage of Labor in Obese Patients: Calling for a New Definition

Tina Bui, Kristina Roloff and Guillermo Valenzuela

Abstract

Obesity is an epidemic worldwide with about half of the population being classified as overweight and obese. Second stage labor arrest may occur more commonly in patients with obesity, leading to a higher number of cesarean deliveries. Second stage arrest is diagnosed based on a fixed time frame without consideration of the total amount of expulsive forces exerted. The beginning of the second stage of labor is determined by an arbitrary parameter that depends on the timing intervals at which patients are examined. In other words, the specific point at which the second stage begins (complete dilation) is influenced by the frequency of examinations conducted during labor. Therefore, it would be reasonable to consider factors such as the cumulative duration of pushing and/or the number of pushes and/or cumulative force generated as clinical measurements to determine the optimal length of the second stage of labor. By redefining the criteria used to define second stage labor dystocia or arrest, we can ensure that patients are given an appropriate amount of time to generate the expulsive forces necessary for a safe vaginal delivery. Here, we will review the evidence to help optimize the management of the second stage.

Keywords: second stage of labor, obesity, maternal body mass index, cesarean delivery, abnormal labor

1. Introduction

The second stage of labor is defined as the time from complete dilation of the cervix to delivery of the fetus. Several factors can influence the length of the second stage, including parity, maternal body mass index (BMI), fetal weight, fetal presentation, fetal position, and the use of analgesia [1]. In this chapter, we will focus on how obesity affects the duration of labor as the prevalence of obesity is rising among reproductive-aged individuals.

Obesity, defined as a BMI ≥ 30 kg/m^2, poses unique challenges for obstetrical providers throughout pregnancy. It increases the risk of hypertensive disorders, gestational diabetes, macrosomia, intrauterine growth restriction, and infections. Intrapartum care of obese women also presents challenges, including a higher rate of cesarean delivery and associated complications such as postoperative wound infections, thromboembolic events, postpartum hemorrhage, endometritis, and delayed wound healing [1]. One study showed the rate of cesarean delivery during the second stage of labor in obese patients was twice as high as that in leaner individuals, especially for those with a BMI ≥ 35 kg/m² [2]. Most of these cesarean deliveries were unscheduled due to labor arrest [2, 3].

Currently, the American College of Obstetricians and Gynecologists (ACOG) and Society for Maternal-Fetal Medicine (SMFM) define second stage of labor arrest as at least 2 hours of pushing in multiparous women and at least 3 hours of pushing in nulliparous women, with longer durations for epidural use and fetal malposition if progress is being documented [4]. However, the actual onset and duration of the second stage can be inaccurately recorded as the very definition of the beginning relies on an arbitrary time point when the examiner finds the cervix to be completely dilated. It would be reasonable to consider the cumulative length of time a patient is pushing, the number of pushes, and/or cumulative force generated as a clinical measurement to define the optimal length of the second stage and potentially change the trigger for diagnosis of second stage labor arrest. This would be a similar concept to using Montevideo units for defining adequate uterine contractility during the first stage of labor.

In this chapter, we will review the evidence on optimal management of the second stage of labor, with a focus on achieving vaginal delivery without increasing maternal and neonatal morbidities and mortalities.

2. Pelvic anatomy and physiology of labor

2.1 Anatomy

The maternal pelvis consists of the bony pelvis and surrounding soft tissue structures. The size and shape of the pelvis play an important role in the second stage of labor. Four different pelvic types have been described (**Figure 1**): gynecoid (41.4%), android (32.5%), anthropoid (23.5%), and platypelloid (2.6%) [5]. The most common pelvic type is gynecoid, which is considered the most favorable shape for fetal descent during the different cardinal movements of labor (engagement, descent, flexion, internal rotation, extension, external rotation). During the second stage of labor, the fetal head is mostly found in an oblique occiput anterior (OA) position [6]. However, certain pelvis types like anthropoid and platypelloid

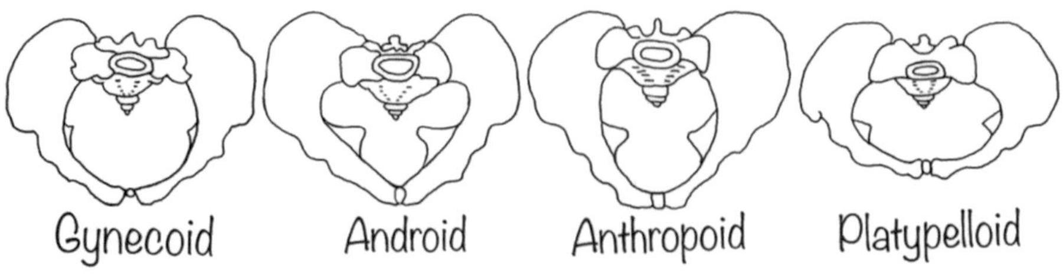

Figure 1.
Illustrating the four different pelvic types, the gynecoid pelvis is considered the most ideal type for childbirth due to its wide pelvic inlet. The android pelvis, more commonly found in males but occasionally in females, has a heart-shaped pelvic inlet with a narrow opening and a pronounced sacrum. The anthropoid pelvis is characterized by an oval-shaped inlet and is often associated with the OP position of the baby's head during labor. Lastly, the platypelloid pelvis is wide and flat in shape.

are at a higher risk of fetal malposition, such as occiput posterior (OP) and occiput transverse (OT) position, respectively. Patients with a fetus in the OP position have been found to have a longer second stage of labor, up to 60 minutes longer compared to a fetus in the OA position [7]. A systematic review of randomized controlled trials demonstrated that manual rotation of the occiput was associated with a higher rate of vaginal delivery: 64.9% in the manual rotation group vs. 59.5% in the control group [8]. Manual rotation also may shorten the second stage of labor by 15 to 30 minutes, depending on parity [8]. Manual rotation causes no difference in neonatal outcomes and thus should be attempted before proceeding to operative delivery or cesarean delivery [4].

2.2 Endocrinology of labor

Hormonal signals play a crucial role in orchestrating the initiation and progression of labor. Throughout pregnancy, progesterone keeps the uterus in a quiescent state [1, 9, 10]. As labor approaches, progesterone levels decline, while estrogen and corticotropin-releasing hormone (CRH) start to rise [9]. CRH is released from the placenta and stimulates the fetal adrenal glands to produce cortisol which in turn boosts the production of prostaglandins [9]. Estrogen also promotes the synthesis of prostaglandins, increases receptivity to oxytocin, and stimulates the growth of uterine muscle, leading to the initiation of labor [9]. Prostaglandins help soften and ripen the cervix [1, 10]. During this time, oxytocin levels and receptors rise, aiding in the stimulation of the smooth muscle fibers in the myometrium leading to an increase in the frequency, duration, and intensity of uterine contractions [9, 10]. Oxytocin is released from the posterior pituitary gland, and its release is regulated by a positive feedback mechanism during labor, where further descent of the fetus into the pelvis increases oxytocin release [6].

3. Second stage of labor

3.1 Current definition of duration of the second stage of labor

The duration of the second stage of labor can vary among individuals and is influenced by several factors. The second stage of labor begins when the cervix is fully dilated and usually last about 50 minutes in nulliparas and 20 minutes in multiparas, however, is increased in duration in patients with epidural analgesia [10]. In 2014, an obstetric care consensus recommended following a specific maximum length to avoid prematurely performing a cesarean delivery: nulliparous with an epidural up to 4 hours, nulliparous without an epidural up to 3 hours, multiparous with an epidural up to 3 hours, and multiparous without an epidural up to 2 hours [4].

3.2 Prolonged second stage of labor

A prolonged second stage of labor refers to a delay in the progression of labor following complete cervical dilation, which has been redefined by ACOG in recent years to prevent primary cesarean sections. Unfortunately, obesity is recognized as one of the leading causes of a protracted labor course, as studies indicate that obese patients take approximately 1.3 hours longer to progress from 4 to 10 cm [1, 11–13]. While it is well-established that the first stage of labor is prolonged in obese patients, the duration of the second stage remains a subject of controversy [13]. Some studies suggest a longer duration [14, 15], others indicate equivalence [16, 17], and others report a shorter duration of the second stage [18]. This variability could be attributed to factors such as the increased likelihood of cesarean delivery interrupting the natural course of labor or the wide range of BMI values encompassed within these studies. Here we approach this issue from a different perspective.

Traditionally, the duration of the second stage of labor is measured in length of time. Defining the start of the second stage based on the cervix reaching 10 cm is prone to inaccuracies due to the variability in frequency of pelvic examination during labor. It is entirely possible that many patients are completely dilated well before the examiner detects it. The length of the second stage also depends on the frequency of uterine contractions, the time a patient spent "laboring down", and any breaks they may take in between or during contractions. Thus, defining a prolonged second stage by the total length of time is confounded by the heterogeneity of the clinical picture. Medical decision-making based on absolute time definitions may even result in patients undergoing cesarean delivery before having an adequate chance or length of time to push. Therefore, we propose using the cumulative length of time a patient is pushing or the number of pushes as a clinical measurement to define the optimal length of the second stage.

Concerns have been raised about the impact of a prolonged second stage of labor on perinatal outcomes. A randomized control trial conducted by Gimovsky et al. demonstrated that an extra hour of pushing reduced the incidence of cesarean delivery from 43.2 to 19.5% without increasing maternal and neonatal morbidity [19]. There have been several studies including a large multicenter randomized control trial, cohort studies, and systematic reviews that have also shown no increase in perinatal outcomes with a prolonged second stage of labor [20–22]. Therefore, it may be reasonable to extend the second stage pushing time for patients without fetal heart rate abnormalities, especially for obese patients [4].

3.3 Uterine contractility

Uterine contractions are essential to descent and ultimately delivery of the fetus. Contractions exhibit three main properties: frequency, duration, and strength [23]. In the second stage of labor, it is observed that contractions last up to 1 minute and recur at intervals no longer than 90 seconds [10]. Obesity is linked to reduced uterine contractility and irregular contraction patterns [11, 14]. While the exact mechanism for dysfunctional contractions in obese patients is unknown, there are several potential causes. *In vitro* myometrial samples from obese patients demonstrate a decrease in intracellular calcium influx during a contraction [11]. Impaired myometrial contractility may also be due to hyperlipidemia in obese patients, as oxytocin receptors are located near cholesterol-rich regions of the cell membrane known as lipid rafts which may be influenced by local lipid accumulation [11].

Despite dysfunctional contractions, obese patients are still capable of generating adequate Montevideo units, but may require higher doses of oxytocin to produce adequate contractions [17]. Obese individuals undergoing labor induction require progressively higher cumulative doses of oxytocin as their BMI class increases [17]. In order to optimize the chances of a vaginal delivery in obese patients, it may be necessary to closely monitor and aggressively adjust oxytocin doses to ensure adequate contractions to facilitate progression of labor.

3.4 Valsalva forces

Expulsive forces, or pushing through cognizant contraction of the striated muscles in the chest and abdomen, have been demonstrated to be necessary for achieving vaginal delivery [24]. Directed pushing, where the patient actively participates and follows verbal instruction, has been associated with a shorter duration of the second stage [6]. It is the cumulative effects of uterine contractions and expulsive forces that are necessary for the fetus to descend through the pelvis, resulting in a vaginal delivery.

We have found that patients with a BMI $\geq$ 35 kg/m^2 generate lower pressure while pushing in the second stage of labor [25]. Lower intrauterine pressure suggests less expulsive force and hence increased risk for second-stage dystocia or arrest. This suggests that obese patients may need a longer second stage of labor to achieve a vaginal birth.

There are several potential explanations for these observations. It is possible that the abdominal musculature in patients with a BMI $\geq$ 35 kg/m^2 is stretched beyond the optimal point of sarcomere overlap and therefore unable to generate adequate expulsive force through muscle contraction. Or perhaps, an increased body weight is also associated with metabolic dysregulation by which hyperlipidemia interferes with calcium influx and leads to fatty infiltration of the muscles, thus impairing abdominal and myometrial contractility. However, further research is needed to explore the exact mechanism.

Since obese patients can not generate sufficient expulsive force per contraction, it may be better to measure the cumulative force of sequential contractions combined with pushing generated during the second stage of labor as a parameter for assessing progress and determining the likelihood of achieving a successful vaginal delivery.

3.5 Immediate versus delay pushing

There are two common practices used in the management of the second stage of labor: (1) delayed pushing, or "laboring down" in which the patient rests and the fetal head passively descends with contractions), and (2) immediate pushing, where pushing with contractions is initiated once the cervix is complete. Delayed pushing was thought to provide several benefits, including reducing maternal fatigue, minimizing the risk of perineal trauma, and allowing time for the baby's head to mold and adjust to the birth canal [26]. However, a meta-analysis of randomized control trials, involving 5445 patients with epidural analgesia, showed delayed pushing was associated with increased morbidity. Among patients in the delayed pushing group, there was a significantly prolonged duration of labor, higher incidence of chorioamnionitis, and lower umbilical cord pH, with no difference in the mode of delivery [27]. Another large multicenter randomized clinical trial including 2414 patients found similar rates of spontaneous vaginal delivery: 85.6% in the immediate pushing group versus 86.5% in the delayed pushing group. Again, in the delayed pushing group there was a longer second stage of labor, higher rates of chorioamnionitis, increase neonatal acidemia, and also higher rates of postpartum hemorrhage [28]. The trial was stopped prematurely because of concern for excess morbidity in the delayed pushing group. Based on these findings, it is reasonable to prioritize immediate pushing over delayed pushing [28].

3.6 Maternal position

There are varying opinions regarding the optimal maternal position during the second stage when pushing. Maternal position may play a significant role in facilitating fetal descent. A Cochrane review comparing different pushing positions found that an upright position offers several benefits, including reduced fetal heart rate abnormalities, decreased rates of episiotomy, and a shorter duration of the second stage of labor by 6.6 minutes [29]. However, an upright position was associated with a higher risk of postpartum hemorrhage when compared to the supine position [29].

Both upright and lateral pushing techniques are effective in preventing perineal trauma [29]. Pushing in the lateral recumbent position can also aid in rotating a fetus in the OP position. In the epidural and position trial collaborative group study, a higher rate of vaginal delivery was observed when patients pushed in a lateral recumbent position compared to other positions [10, 32]. Nevertheless, due to the variability in findings and individual patient and provider preference, there is no position recommended over others.

ACOG recommends frequent position changes during labor to enhance comfort and promote optimal fetal positioning, as long as these positions are not contraindicated for the patient [30]. It is important for healthcare providers to consider individual circumstances, patient preferences, and safety when determining the most appropriate pushing position.

3.7 Operative vaginal delivery

Over the last 15 years, the rate of operative vaginal deliveries has declined as the rates of cesarean deliveries rise [4]. An operative vaginal delivery involves the use of either a vacuum or forceps to assist in the delivery of the baby. This procedure may be necessary in situations where there is a need to expedite delivery due to maternal or fetal factors. Some specific indications for operative vaginal delivery include a prolonged second stage of labor, non-reassuring fetal heart tones, maternal exhaustion, and maternal cardiopulmonary disorders or brain aneurysms that prevent prolonged maternal pushing [23].

Although there are risks associated with operative vaginal delivery, including maternal perineal trauma, lacerations, fetal scalp and skull injuries, and intracranial hemorrhages, large studies have demonstrated no difference in serious neonatal morbidity between operative vaginal delivery and unplanned cesarean delivery [4]. The safety of the procedure depends on the practitioner's experience and the station of the presenting part [32]. The overall success rate of operative vaginal delivery has been reported to be between 86 and 91% [33]. However, lower success rates have been found in cases where maternal BMI exceeds 30 kg/m^2 and ironically, maternal obesity is known to be a risk factor for operative vaginal deliveries [31, 34].

Because obese patients generate lower pressure during pushing, an operative device may be needed to supplement the force during the second stage of labor.

Overall, the decision to proceed with an operative vaginal delivery is based on individual circumstances and requires careful consideration of the potential benefits and risks for both the mother and the fetus. It is important for healthcare providers to assess each situation on a case-by-case basis to make an informed decision, but operative vaginal deliveries should be considered a safe and acceptable alternative to cesarean delivery [4].

4. Pain control

4.1 Epidural analgesia

Epidural analgesia use in labor is a popular choice for pain relief among many individuals due to its effectiveness. However, the use of epidural analgesia has an impact on the progression of labor. A meta-analysis revealed that epidural anesthesia prolongs the second stage of labor by approximately 15 to 28 minutes [35], which means that patients who opt for epidural analgesia are typically given more time to complete the second stage of labor.

Additionally, studies have explored the impact of the timing of epidural administration by comparing an early versus late epidural placement. Despite some controversies, the collective findings indicate that the timing of epidural placement has minimal impact on the overall progression of labor [36]. However, a recent study of 7647 patients demonstrated an association between early epidural use (< 6 cm) and a decreased risk of a prolonged second stage of labor [37]. Based on these findings, it is reasonable to consider epidural use at any point during labor, taking into account the patient's personal values and preferences.

It is worth noting that alternative pain control options, such as intravenous and intramuscular opioids, are available but are generally recognized to be less effective than epidural analgesia, and are avoided during the second stage of labor due to concern for respiratory depression of the neonate.

5. Conclusion

Optimizing the management of the second stage of labor involves considering factors such as pelvic shape and size, fetal position and presentation, Montevideo units, Valsalva forces, timing of pushing, maternal position, and considering operative vaginal deliveries when appropriate. Optimal, evidence-based practice recommendations include:

- Ensuring adequate Montevideo units, particularly in obese patients who are more prone to dysfunctional labor.

- Initiating immediate pushing at the time of completion, irrespective of the use of epidural analgesia or the urge to push.

- Attempting manual rotation of a fetus from an occiput posterior or occiput transverse position to an occiput anterior position.

- Encouraging patients to follow their instinct to bear down when they feel the urge to do so, in a position they find comfortable

It is important to appreciate that an unplanned and emergent cesarean section during second stage of labor is associated with a significantly increased maternal and perinatal morbidity and mortality [38]. Therefore, every attempt should be made to achieve a safe vaginal birth. To facilitate this goal, it may be necessary to redefine the optimal length of the second stage of labor, considering alternative clinical measurements such as the cumulative length of time a patient spends pushing, the number of pushes, and/or the cumulative force generated.

Lastly, it is important to note that obesity presents numerous challenges throughout pregnancy, and these challenges may become more pronounced in the second stage of labor. Ultimately, the most effective strategy for minimizing complications during pregnancy and delivery is the prevention of obesity itself and achieving adequate weight loss prior to conception.

Acknowledgements

We have no acknowledgements.

Conflict of interest

The authors declare no conflict of interest.

Author details

Tina Bui*, Kristina Roloff and Guillermo Valenzuela
Department of Women's Health, Arrowhead Regional Medical Center, Colton, USA

*Address all correspondence to: tmbui04@gmail.com

References

[1] Creasy RK, Resnik R, Greene MF, Iams JD, Lockwood CJ. Creasy and Resnik's Maternal-Fetal Medicine: Principles and Practice. Seventh ed. Philadelphia: Elsevier/Saunders; 2014. p. 1282

[2] Maged AM, Belal DS, Marie HM, Rashwan H, Abdelaziz S, Gabr AA, et al. Prospective study of the effect of maternal body mass index on labor progress in nulliparous women in Egypt. International Journal of Gynaecology and Obstetrics. 2017;**139**:329-335. DOI: 10.1002/ijgo.12322

[3] Cedergren MI. Non-elective caesarean delivery due to ineffective uterine contractility or due to obstructed labour in relation to maternal body mass index. European Journal of Obstetrics, Gynecology, and Reproductive Biology. 2009;**145**:163-166. DOI: 10.1016/j.ejogrb.2009.05.022

[4] American College of Obstetricians and Gynecologists (College); Society for Maternal-Fetal Medicine, Caughey AB, Cahill AG, Guise JM, Rouse DJ. Safe prevention of the primary cesarean delivery. American Journal of Obstetrics and Gynecology. 2014;**210**:179-193. DOI: 10.1016/j.ajog.2014.01.026

[5] Siccardia MA, Imonugo O, Arbor TC, Valle C. Anatomy, Abdomen and Pelvis, Pelvic Inlet. Treasure Island: StatPearls Publishing; 2022

[6] Hofmeyr GJ, Singata-Madliki M. The second stage of labor. Best Practice & Research. Clinical Obstetrics & Gynaecology. 2020;**67**:53-64. DOI: 10.1016/j.bpobgyn.2020.03.012

[7] Cheng Y, Shaffer B, Caughey A. The second stage of labor and persistent occiput posterior position: Patient or intervention? American Journal of Obstetrics and Gynecology. 2013;**208**:237-386. DOI: 10.1016/j.ajog.2012.10.507

[8] Bertholdt C, Morel O, Zuily S, Ambroise-Grandjean G. Manual rotation of occiput posterior or transverse positions: A systematic review and meta-analysis of randomized controlled trials. American Journal of Obstetrics and Gynecology. 2022;**226**:781-793. DOI: 10.1016/j.ajog.2021.11.033

[9] Buckley SJ. Executive summary of hormonal physiology of childbearing: Evidence and implications for women, babies, and maternity care. The Journal of Perinatal Education. 2015;**24**:145-153. DOI: 10.1891/1058-1243.24.3.145

[10] Cunningham F, Leveno KJ, Dashe JS, Hoffman BL, Spong CY, Casey BM. Williams Obstetrics. 26th ed. New York: McGraw Hill; 2022. p. 2049

[11] Chin JR, Henry E, Holmgren CM, Varner MW, Branch DW. Maternal obesity and contraction strength in the first stage of labor. American Journal of Obstetrics and Gynecology. 2012;**207**(129):e1-e6. DOI: 10.1016/j.ajog.2012.06.044

[12] Carlhall S, Kallen K, Blomberg M. Maternal body mass index and duration of labor. European Journal of Obstetrics, Gynecology, and Reproductive Biology. 2013;**171**:49-53. DOI: 10.1016/j.ejogrb.2013.08.021

[13] Gimovsky AC. Defining arrest in the first and second stages of labor. Minerva Obstetrics and Gynecology. 2021;**73**:6-18. DOI: 10.23736/S2724-606X.20.04644-4

[14] Zhang J, Bricker L, Wray S, Quenby S. Poor uterine contractility in obese women. BJOG : An International Journal of Obstetrics and Gynaecology. 2007;**114**:343-348. DOI: 10.1111/j.1471-0528.2006.01233.x

[15] Buhimschi CS, Buhimschi IA, Malinow AM, Kopelman JN, Weiner CP. Pushing in labor: Performance and not endurance. American Journal of Obstetrics and Gynecology. 2002;**186**:1339-1344. DOI: 10.1067/mob.2002.122402

[16] Buhimschi CS, Buhimschi IA, Malinow AM, Weiner CP. Intrauterine pressure during the second stage of labor in obese women. Obstetrics and Gynecology. 2004;**103**:225-230. DOI: 10.1097/01.AOG.0000102706.84063.C7

[17] Roloff K, Peng S, Sanchez-Ramos L, Valenzuela GJ. Cumulative oxytocin dose during induction of labor according to maternal body mass index. International Journal of Gynaecology and Obstetrics. 2015;**131**:54-58. DOI: 10.1016/j.ijgo.2015.04.038

[18] Ellekjaer KL, Bergholt T, Lokkegaard E. Maternal obesity and its effect on labour duration in nulliparous women: A retrospective observational cohort study. BMC Pregnancy and Childbirth. 2017;**17**:222. DOI: 10.1002/ijgo.12322

[19] Gimovsky A, Berghella V. Randomized controlled trial of prolonged second stage: Extending time limit vs usual guidelines. American Journal of Obstetrics and Gynecology. 2016;**214**:361.e1-361.e6. DOI: 10.1016/j.ajog.2015.12.042

[20] Rouse DJ, Weiner SJ, Bloom SL, Varner MW, Spong CY, Ramin SM, et al. Eunice Kennedy Shriver National Institute of child health, human development maternal-fetal medicine units network. Second-stage labor duration in nulliparous women: Relationship to maternal and perinatal outcomes. American Journal of Obstetrics and Gynecology. 2009;**201**(357):e1-e7. DOI: 10.1016/j.ajog.2009.08.003

[21] Young C, Bhattacharya S, Woolner A, Ingram A, Smith N, Raja EA, et al. Maternal and perinatal outcomes of prolonged second stage of labour: A historical cohort study of over 51,000 women. BMC Pregnancy and Childbirth. 2023;**23**:467. DOI: 10.1186/s12884-023-05733-z

[22] Altman MR, Lydon-Rochelle MT. Prolonged second stage of labor and risk of adverse maternal and perinatal outcomes: A systematic review. Birth. 2006;**33**:315-322. DOI: 10.1111/j.1523-536X.2006.00129.x

[23] Oikonomou M, Chandraharan E. Management of the second stage of labor. In: Chandraharan E, editor. The Continuous Textbook of Women's Medicine Series – Obstetrics Module. Vol. 11. London: Glown; 2021. DOI: 10.3843/GLOWM.415143

[24] Bansal R, Goyal MK, Modi M. Management of myasthenia gravis during pregnancy. Indian Journal of Pharmacology. 2018;**50**:302-308. DOI: 10.4103/ijp.IJP_452_17

[25] Bui T, Witcik K, Roloff K, Novack M, Valenzuela GJ. Intra-abdominal uterine pressure during the second stage of labor according to body mass index. In: Poster Session Presented at: Pacific Coast Obstetrical and Gynecological Annual Meeting. Maui, Hawaii: PCOGS; 2022 August 31 – 4 September

[26] Fraser WD, Marcoux S, Krauss I, Douglas J, Goulet C, Boulvain M. Multicenter, randomized, controlled trial of delayed pushing for nulliparous women in the second stage of labor with continuous epidural analgesia. The PEOPLE (pushing early or pushing late with epidural) study group. American Journal of Obstetrics and Gynecology. 2000;**182**:1165-1172. DOI: 10.1067/mob.2000.105197

[27] Di Mascio D, Saccone G, Bellussi F, Al-Kouatly HB, Brunelli R, Benedetti Panici P, et al. Delayed versus immediate pushing in the second stage of labor in women with neuraxial analgesia: A systematic review and meta-analysis of randomized controlled trials. American Journal of Obstetrics and Gynecology. 2020;**223**:189-203. DOI: 10.1016/j.ajog.2020.02.002

[28] Cahill AG, Srinivas SK, Tita ATN, Caughey AB, Richter HE, Gregory WT, et al. Effect of immediate vs delayed pushing on rates of spontaneous vaginal delivery among nulliparous women receiving Neuraxial analgesia: A randomized clinical trial. Journal of the American Medical Association. 2018;**320**:1444-1454. DOI: 10.1001/jama.2018.13986

[29] Huang J, Zang Y, Ren LH, Li FJ, Lu H. A review and comparison of common maternal positions during the second-stage of labor. The International Journal of Nursing Sciences. 2019;**6**:460-467. DOI: 10.1016/j.ijnss.2019.06.007

[30] Epidural and Position Trial Collaborative Group. Upright versus lying down position in second stage of labour in nulliparous women with low dose epidural: BUMPES randomised controlled trial. BMJ. 2017;**359**:j4471. DOI: 10.1136/bmj.j4471

[31] ACOG Committee Opinion No. 766. Approaches to limit intervention during labor and birth. Obstetrics and Gynecology. 2019;**133**:e164-e173. DOI: 10.1097/AOG.0000000000003074

[32] Feeley C, Crossland N, Betran AP, Weeks A, Downe S, Kingdon C. Training and expertise in undertaking assisted vaginal delivery (AVD): A mixed methods systematic review of practitioners views and experiences. Reproductive Health. 2021;**18**:92. DOI: 10.1186/s12978-021-01146-3

[33] Martin I, Ayres-de-Campos D. Assisted vaginal delivery in obese women. In: Mahmood T, Lim CC, editors. Handbook of Obesity in Obstetrics and Gynecology. Cambridge: Academic Press; 2023. pp. 353-356. DOI: 10.1016/B978-0-323-89904-8.00020-2

[34] Faucett AM, Metz TD. Delivery of the obese gravida. Clinical Obstetrics and Gynecology. 2016;**59**:180-192. DOI: 10.1097/GRF.0000000000000175

[35] Meng ML, Smiley R. Modern Neuraxial anesthesia for labor and delivery. F1000Res. 2017;**6**:1211. DOI: 10.12688/f1000research.11130.1

[36] Sng BL, Leong WL, Zeng Y, Siddiqui FJ, Assam PN, Lim Y, et al. Early versus late initiation of epidural analgesia for labour. Cochrane Database of Systematic Reviews. 2014;**10**:CD007238. DOI: 10.1002/14651858.CD007238.pub2

[37] Lewkowitz AK, Tuuli MG, Stout MJ, Woolfolk C, Roehl K, Macones GA, et al. Epidurals and the modern labor curve: How epidural timing impacts Fetal Station during active labor. American Journal of Perinatology. 2018;**35**:421-426. DOI: 10.1055/s-0037-1617457

[38] Pergialiotis V, Vlachos DG, Rodolakis A, Haidopoulos D, Thomakos N, Vlachos GD. First versus second stage C/S maternal and neonatal morbidity: A systematic review and meta-analysis. European Journal of Obstetrics, Gynecology, and Reproductive Biology. 2014;**175**:15-24. DOI: 10.1016/j.ejogrb.2013.12.033

Section 3

Neonatal Outcome

Chapter 4

Assesment of Sign and Symptoms Stunting Wasting Risk of Newborn in the Perinatal

Suryani Manurung

Abstract

The scope of this topic is the measurement and assessment of newborns and infants under 2 years of age with the risk of stunting and wasting. This book was compiled in an effort to facilitate the handling of stunting. The topic of stunting is discussed in this book according to trend issues that are widely discussed globally. Apart from being a global issue, we also see the impact of stunting which can hamper children's intelligence. The information presented in this book is how to detect the risk of stunting and wasting through an assessment of signs and symptoms. Any data obtained from the results of the assessment becomes evidence-based evidence to be used in overcoming the causes of stunting and wasting through interventions that will be given to the baby later. Then monitor the baby's development in the next year's life period. This book was prepared by adopting information from previous research and needs to be published as a guideline for health workers to prevent babies from experiencing the risk of stunting and wasting.

Keywords: assessment, measurement, newborn, perinatal, stunting

1. Introduction

Stunting is a picture of growth and development disorders in children and is one of the causes of stunted children's height. Study results from UNICEF (2020) Indonesia is one of the countries with the highest cases of stunting and wasting among children in the world. The result of a basic health survey, in Indonesia in 2007 the prevalence of stunting was 36.8%. The majority of stunting toddlers increased in 2013 to 37.2%. In the 2018 survey, the prevalence of stunting in children under 2 years of age was 29.9%. In toddlers, by 30.8% [1]. Then in 2019, the prevalence of stunting was 27.67% [2]. Before COVID-19, Indonesia was already facing high levels of malnutrition. Then during the COVID-19 period, malnutrition in children under five experienced an increase in the impact of a declining family economy. This condition affects child morbidity and mortality related to malnutrition. Currently, more than two million children are severely underweight, and more than seven million children under the age of 5 are stunted [3]. Globally, editing is also a case that is currently being discussed.

Several countries have overcome stunting based on data found from current cases. Urgent action to prevent and reduce the problem of stunting and wasting with an evidence-based approach. Identification of signs and symptoms of stunting risk in newborns is carried out at the best time, namely early in pregnancy and after delivery. So a preventive approach to overcome the risk of stunting and wasting needs to be considered in the perinatal period, namely pregnancy to delivery [4]. It is hoped that fetuses in the womb who are at high risk of experiencing stunting and wasting can be detected early, so that after birth interventions can be carried out according to the triggering factors. The role of the mother is a key factor in preventing stunting and wasting. The mother is the only source of nutrition for the developing child during the critical period of 1000 days, the first 6 months of a baby's life through exclusive breastfeeding [5]. Then evaluate the development of stunting risk in newborns for the following year with anthropometric assessments and clinical nutritional assessments. The book that will be compiled outlines the elements that will be identified in assessing babies at risk of stunting and wasting.

The scope of this topic is the assessment of newborns and infants under 2 years of age with the risk of stunting and wasting. This book was compiled in an effort to facilitate the handling of stunting. The topic of stunting is discussed in this book according to trend issues that are widely discussed globally. Apart from being a global issue, we also see the impact of stunting which can hamper children's intelligence. The information presented in this book is how to detect the risk of stunting and wasting through an assessment of signs and symptoms. Any data obtained from the results of the assessment becomes evidence-based evidence to be used in overcoming the causes of stunting and wasting through interventions that will be given to the baby later. Then monitor the baby's development in the next year's life period. This book was prepared by adopting information from previous research and needs to be published as a guideline for health workers to prevent babies from experiencing the risk of stunting and wasting.

2. Overview of stunting and wasting

Malnutrition is expressed in the form of stunting and wasting. These two problems often appear together as a form of malnutrition in the same population. There are several findings that illustrate that wasting and stunting have many of the same causative factors [6]. Wasting is described as a condition that tends to look too thin for a person's height, or in terms of weight for height. Wasting due to food shortages and/or acute illness [6]. Stunting can occur in the womb and continue for the first 2 years of life after birth [7].

Stunting is an indication of chronic malnutrition, which is illustrated by a short body structure. Features of wasting and stunting, for example, children under 5 years of age have low weight for age (stunting) and low weight for height (wasting). This indicator can be considered an indicator of malnutrition [6]. Thus WHO defines stunting as growth retardation where the child's weight is less than −2 SD of the z score for height or weight-for-height Z-scores (WHZ), height/length for age (length-for-age z score) (HAZ) [8]. Stunting can affect a child's development process starting from conception to after birth in the third or fourth year of life [6].

The incidence of detected babies experiencing stunting is related to pregnancy and postpartum [9]. Several prenatal factors include maternal anemia during pregnancy, nutritional variations, knowledge during pregnancy, family economy, accompanying diseases, and infections. All of these factors are associated with the incidence of stunting in newborns [9, 10]. Malnutrition in cases of stunting includes inadequate maternal nutrition, intrauterine malnutrition, lack/not breastfeeding until 6 months of age, delay in introduction and provision of complementary foods, inadequate complementary foods (quantity and quality), and impaired absorption of nutrients due to disease infectious or digestive. Likewise, births related to stunting, namely babies born at a premature age [9]. During the postpartum period, the mother's knowledge and education related to stunting [11].

The critical window (sensitive period) for fetal growth and development is expressed as the critical period, i.e. from the intrauterine period and early after birth [12]. The period from conception to the second year after birth (first thousand days) is a critical window for intervention. The period of intrauterine growth of the brain experiences rapid development, which will describe the physical characteristics and abilities of a person in the next life. To maintain brain growth, environmental conditions, and atmosphere during the critical window period are moments that need to be considered so that postpartum wasting and stunting do not occur until the following year.

Stunting with chronic malnutrition is associated with structural and functional pathologies of the brain [7]. Chronic nutritional deficiency causes damage to the brain's nerve tissue, which affects the growth and development of children. So that chronic malnutrition triggers stunting accompanied by disturbances, and cognitive delays during infancy, childhood, and adolescence. The description of the delay can be measured in growth and development according to the child's age group, namely three to 5 years, and differences in cognitive abilities [13]. The syndrome of stunting tends to occur more frequently in developing countries. Where the per capita income of the family does not yet have the ability to provide sufficient nutrition for pregnant women and newborns [13]. In connection with this crisis, health workers and the public need to be facilitated with information in assessing the signs and symptoms of newborns who are at risk of stunting.

3. Stunting syndrome determinants

The term determinant of health is used synonymously with risk factors. In the context of health policy, determinants are defined as health risks that are general, abstract, related to inequality, and difficult to control by individuals. Abstract understanding is then presented in an operational form. Determine stunting syndrome is a set of risk factors that can be used to predict the size of the risk of stunting that might occur. In this case, quoted from several sources, there are 20 predictors of the risk of stunting. The twenty predictors are categorized into 4 groups namely (1) household and housing characteristics; (2) characteristics of mother and father; (3) antenatal care services, and (4) child characteristics [4]. The following is the relationship between risk predictors for stunting (**Figure 1**).

First, determinants based on household and housing, namely: number of family members, number of children under five, fuel for cooking, source of drinking water, toilet facilities, and family income. Both are determinants of the characteristics of the mother and father. Consists of education, employment status, and mother's age at birth. The third antenatal care service consists of the number of visits to pregnant women and the number of iron/folic acid supplements consumed during pregnancy. The four determinants of child characteristics consist of the sex of the child, the child's

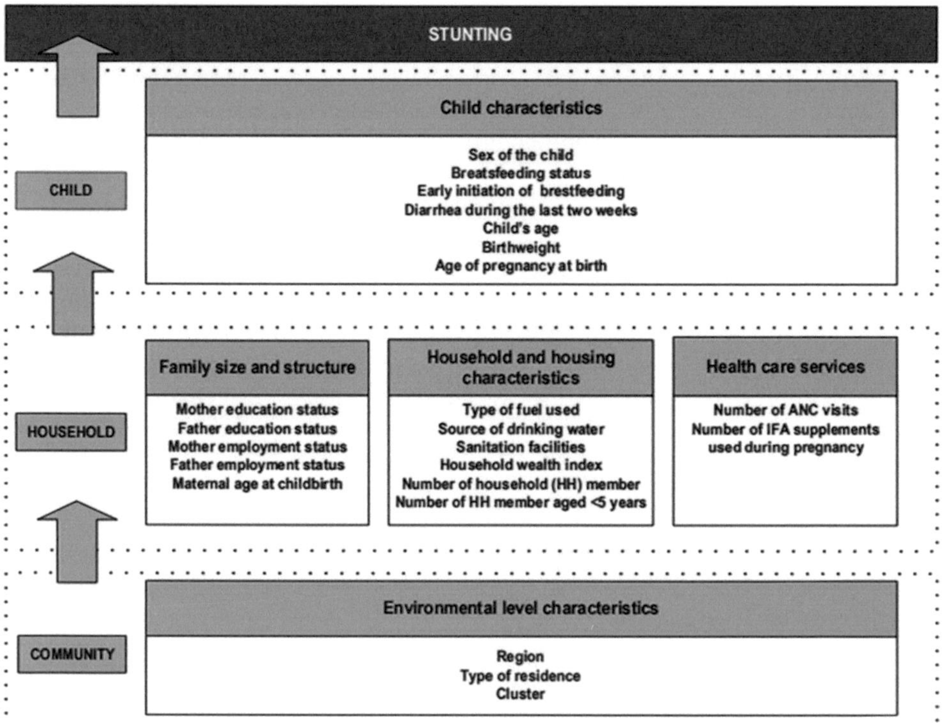

Figure 1.
The relationship between the characteristics of stunting predictors (Source: Titaley et al. [4]).

weight at birth, gestational age at delivery, past breastfeeding, time to start breastfeeding the baby after birth, history of diarrhea during the last 2 weeks, and the child's age when studied.

Based on the test results of the stunting predictor, it shows that the determinant predictor of stunting has a relationship to the incidence of stunting in several areas when applied both in cities and in villages [4]. Testing of the quality of the determinants of stunting syndrome is applied to a wide area of coverage. The data obtained was stated to be representative of the population and to be able to describe the incidence of stunting in that one area. Collection of stunting data with determinants of stunting can be used as a foundation in formulating a policy decision. This policy decision helps design an effective evidence-based intervention to reduce the prevalence of stunting in children under 2 years of age in Indonesia, particularly in the perinatal period [14].

4. Measurement instrument stunting, wasting syndrome

Decision-making on the incidence of stunting and wasting syndrome begins with gathering information on risk factors. So that the data collected in concluding the problem of stunting and wasting are supported by comprehensive data and interventions that will be taken according to the triggering factors. Information obtained from risk factors is supported by data obtained from mothers and family members. The assessment tools collected from previous research for risk factors are as follows: [4, 14].

4.1 Risk factor data collection

Instructions for accessing all information related to risk factors for stunting syndrome and wasting that must be collected:

4.1.1 Household and housing conditions

Information that needs to be collected regarding the risk of stunting and wasting for household and housing conditions, namely:

- Number of family members living together in one house (identifying all family members in reducing the risk of infection transmission)
- The size of the house occupied (Identify the eligibility of the residence divided by the number of occupants and the risk of other sources of infection)
- Number of children under five in the family (identify the amount of costs as well as duties and responsibilities that must be fulfilled by the family to maintain family health, especially children under five).
- Facilities for the use of fuel in cooking (identifying the risk of sources of pollution for respiratory problems that can physically aggravate children under five or pregnant women)
- Consumption of drinking water sources (identifying the availability of drinking water needs for consumption that meets health)
- Availability of washing and toilet facilities (identifying sources of risk of infection that may impact the baby's health problems)
- Family income in one month (identifying the financial ability to meet household needs and consumption of nutrition for each household member, especially toddlers)

4.1.2 Characteristics of mother and father

Information that needs to be collected regarding the risk of stunting and wasting on the characteristics of mothers and fathers, namely:

- Parent education (identifying the level of education, good education facilitates good knowledge, can more easily reach and evaluate the health status of family members and toddlers, especially in terms of nutritional status)
- Parents' work status (identifying parents' work can find out the time spent by parents in caring for toddlers and the number of finances earned in meeting household needs and toddlers' nutritional needs)
- Maternal age at delivery (identifying risk factors that affect the health of toddlers in the womb)

- Parents' cultural traditions (identifying traditions that deviate from health principles so that they have the potential to trigger toddlers to experience illness) [15].

4.1.3 Prenatal care services

Information that needs to be collected regarding the risk of stunting and wasting for antenatal care services, namely:

- Number of visits for pregnant women (Implementation of ANC is highly recommended at least eight (8) times for each pregnant woman to reduce the incidence of death during pregnancy and childbirth. ANC visits can identify risk factors and comorbidities during pregnancy as early as possible so as not to interfere with fetal growth and development intrauterine. So that the risk of experiencing stunting and wasting after birth can be overcome)

- The amount of iron/folic acid supplements consumed during pregnancy (Fe element is the most important element for the formation of red blood cells. So pregnant women are required to consume a minimum of 60 tablets of Fe during their pregnancy to prevent anemia and nutritional intake for the fetus while in the womb Folic acid reduces free radicals that can interfere with fetal growth).

4.1.4 Child characteristics

Information that needs to be collected regarding the risk of stunting and wasting for children's characteristics, namely:

- The sex of the child (there is no difference in the sex of the child for stunting, but it is necessary to study the differences in child care according to the preferred sex in one tribe) [16].

- Child's weight at birth. (The risk of stunting can be seen from the child's weight at birth with a history of maternal weight gain during small pregnancies) [16, 17].

- Gestational age at delivery (identifies gestational age at delivery as an indicator of stunting risk) [18].

- Duration of breastfeeding (One of the causes of stunting, and wasting is a history of exclusive breastfeeding. Previous information stated that toddlers who receive exclusive breastfeeding have a lower risk of experiencing stunting and wasting. Exclusive breastfeeding provides a protective effect against stunting in infants [15, 19].

- Time to start breastfeeding the baby after birth (breastfeeding that starts immediately after birth (IMD/early initiation of breastfeeding), provides coverage of the baby's nutrition and immunity) [15].

- History of diarrhea during the last 2 weeks when reviewed (identifying poor hygiene practices in families that have an impact on diarrhea in infants and can reduce the immune system of babies who are stunted, wasted, and those who are not stunted) [20].

- Age of the child at the time of the study (identifying the age of the child under five at risk of stunting for follow-up in anthropometric measurements).

4.2 Physical examination of nutritional status at risk of stunting and wasting

The nutritional status of newborn babies can be determined based on their height and weight. Measurement of the height and weight of newborns using anthropometric standards. Interpretation of height and weight based on anthropometric standards identifies the risk of stunting, wasting or obesity. Anthropometry is a standard for measuring the nutritional status of babies under 5 years of age. This standard has been socialized to health workers in primary to tertiary health services. Height and weight checks can be applied universally at all ages, including pregnant women. Measuring the weight and height of the uterine fundus of pregnant women can determine the nutritional status of pregnant women and interpret the weight of the fetus in the womb. Low fetal weight in the womb can cause the baby to experience low weight after birth. So identifying measurements of a baby's height and weight after birth is very precise in identifying the risk of stunting and wasting.

4.2.1 Anthropometric measurements

Anthropometric measurements use index weight for height, height for age, weight for age, and other indices such as weight gain for pregnant women. (WHO, 1995) The anthropometric standards for children in Indonesia refer to the WHO Child Growth Standards for children aged 0–5 years. (Mentri Kesehatan Republik Indonesia, 2020) Anthropometric standard sizes for infants aged 0 (zero) to 60 (sixty) months in identifying categories of nutritional problems, one of which is the index of weight according to body length or height (WB/BL or WB/HB). The category index is malnutrition (severely wasted); malnutrition (wasted); good nutrition (normal); more nutritional risk (possible risk of overweight); more nutrition (overweight); obesity (obese).(Mentri Kesehatan Republik Indonesia, 2020).

Another physical examination in measuring nutritional status uses the Waterlow classification. Measurement of body weight for height or weight-for-height Z-scores (WHZ) adapted according to the Waterlow classification consists of (1) WHZ low (stunting and wasting at the same time) (2) WHZ normal (stunting only) (3) WHZ high (Short stature with excess weight appear side by side). (Ferreira, 2020) Medium The size value is usually expressed in the form of a z-score. Height-for-age z-score, (HAZ) is in measuring stunting.

The following is a physical examination to detect the risk of stunting and wasting based on anthropometry and clinical assessment nutrition (CAN score).

4.3 Clinical assessment of the nutritional status of the newborn

4.3.1 Anthropometric neonatal

Measurement of body weight/weight-for-height z score (WHZ) or measurement of height-for-age/height/length-for-age z score (HAZ) (**Table 1**).

The classification of nutritional status is adapted from Waterlow. The difference between stunting and wasting is based on measurements of body weight and height. Wasting is a low weight-for-height z score (WHZ). Stunting is defined as a low height/length-for-age z score (HAZ). (Ferreira, 2020).

Here is a table for detecting wasting based on gender.

Description of **Tables 2–5** Measurement of body weight-for-height Z-scores (WHZ) for children adapted according to the Waterlow classification consists of (1) WHZ low stunting and wasting at the same time) (2) WHZ normal (stunting only) (3) WHZ high (Short stature with excess weight appears side by side) [21]. Interpretation of the value of the size of the height-for-age z-score, (HAZ) explains stunting

Nutritional condition	**HAZ (SD)**		**WHZ (SD)**	
	Normal (≥ - 2)	**Low** (< - 2)	**Normal** (≥ -2 to ≤2)	**Low** (< -2)
Eutrophy	V		V	
Chronic undernutrition (stunting)		V	V	
Acute undernutrition (wasting)	V			V
Decompensated chronic undernutrition[a]		V		V
Overweight				
Short stature with overweight				
Total				

[a]*Concurrently wasting and stunting.*
This table describes the six categories defined as indicators of nutritional conditions, namely: eutrophic (normal height and weight), acute undernutrition (wasting), chronic undernutrition (stunting), decompensated chronic undernutrition, Overweight.

Table 1.
Anthropometric assessment of the nutritional status of children: a new approach based on an adaptation of the Waterlow classification [21].

Body Length (CM)	Body Weight (Kg)						
	-3 SD	-2 SD	-1SD	Median	+1SD	+2 SD	+3 SD
45.0	1.9	2.0	2.2	2.4	2.7	3.0	3.3
45.5	1.9	2.1	2.3	2.5	2.8	3.1	3.4
46.0	2.0	2.2	2.4	2.6	2.9	3.1	3.5
46.5	2.1	2.3	2.5	2.7	3.0	3.2	3.6
47.0	2.1	2.3	2.5	2.8	3.0	3.3	3.7
47.5	2.2	2.4	2.6	2.9	3.1	3.4	3.8
48.0	2.3	2.5	2.7	2.9	3.2	3.6	3.9
48.5	2.3	2.6	2.8	3.0	3.3	3.7	4.0
49.0	2.4	2.6	2.9	3.1	3.4	3.8	4.2
49.5	2.5	2.7	3.0	3.2	3.5	3.9	4.3
50.0	2.6	2.8	3.0	3.3	3.6	4.0	4.4
50.5	2.7	2.9	3.1	3.4	3.8	4.1	4.5
51.0	2.7	3.0	3.2	3.5	3.9	4.2	4.7
51.5	2.8	3.1	3.3	3.6	4.0	4.4	4.8
52.0	2.9	3.2	3.5	3.8	4.1	4.5	5.0
52.5	3.0	3.3	3.6	3.9	4.2	4.6	5.1
53.0	3.1	3.4	3.7	4.0	4.4	4.8	5.3
53.5	3.2	3.5	3.8	4.1	4.5	4.9	5.4

54.0	3.3	3.6	3.9	4.3	4.7	5.1	5.6
54.5	3.4	3.7	4.0	4.4	4.8	5.3	5.8
55.0	3.6	3.8	4.2	4.5	5.0	5.4	6.0
55.5	3.7	4.0	4.3	4.7	5.1	5.6	6.1
56.0	3.8	4.1	4.4	4.8	5.3	5.8	6.3
56.5	3.9	4.2	4.6	5.0	5.4	5.9	6.5
57.0	4.0	4.3	4.7	5.1	5.6	6.1	6.7
57.5	4.1	4.5	4.9	5.3	5.7	6.3	6.9
58.0	4.3	4.6	5.0	5.4	5.9	6.4	7.1
58.5	4.4	4.7	5.1	5.6	6.1	6.6	7.2
59.0	4.5	4.8	5.3	5.7	6.2	6.8	7.4
59.5	4.6	5.0	5.4	5.9	6.4	7.0	7.6
60.0	4.7	5.1	5.4	6.0	6.5	7.1	7.8
60.5	4.8	5.2	5.6	6.1	6.7	7.3	8.0
61.0	4.9	5.3	5.8	6.3	6.8	7.4	8.1
61.5	5.0	5.4	5.9	6.4	7.0	7.6	8.3
62.0	5.1	5.6	6.0	6.5	7.1	7.7	8.5
62.5	5.2	5.7	6.1	6.7	7.2	7.9	8.6
63.0	5.3	5.8	6.2	6.8	7.4	8.0	8.8
63.5	5.4	5.9	6.4	6.9	7.5	8.2	8.9
64.0	5.5	6.0	6.5	7.0	7.6	8.3	9.1
64.5	5.6	6.1	6.6	7.1	7.8	8.5	9.3
65.0	5.7	6.2	6.7	7.3	7.9	8.6	9.4
65.5	5.8	6.3	6.8	7.4	8.0	8.7	9.6
66.0	5.9	6.4	6.9	7.5	8.2	8.9	9.7
66.5	6.0	6.5	7.0	7.6	8.3	9.0	9.9
67.0	6.1	6.6	7.1	7.7	8.4	9.2	10.0
67.5	6.2	6.7	7.2	7.9	8.5	9.3	10.2
68.0	6.3	6.8	7.3	8.0	8.7	9.4	10.3
68.5	6.4	6.9	7.5	8.1	8.8	9.6	10.5
69.0	6.5	7.0	7.6	8.2	8.9	9.7	10.6
69.5	6.6	7.1	7.7	8.3	9.0	9.8	10.8
70.0	6.6	7.2	7.8	8.4	9.2	10.0	10.9

This table describes describe the standard weight according to body length (weight/l height) based on the threshold (Z-Score) for boys to be declared: severely wasted (< -3 SD), wasted (-3 SD to < -2 SD), good nutrition (-2SD to +1SD), possible risk of overweight (> +1 SD to +2SD), Obese (>+3SD).

Table 2.
Standard weight-for-height z score boys aged [22].

with a value HAZ low in chronic undernutrition (stunting), decompensated chronic undernutrition (stunting dan wasting).

4.4 Clinical nutritional assessment (CAN)

4.4.1 Hair

The condition of the hair is assessed by four indicators. Indicator 1. There is a space on the head where hair does not grow, hair is straight and straight, hair pigmentation is reduced, and hair is gathered together. Indicator 2: thick, straight thin hair and more hair growth. Indicator 3: thick hair, sparse growth, few straight hairs. Indicator 4: hair is thick, dense, smooth, shiny, and easy to comb.

4.4.2 Cheek

The structure and texture of the cheeks are assessed by four indicators. Indicator (1). There is almost no fat structure on the cheeks, the face is narrow. (2). The structure of the cheek pads is significantly reduced (3). The cushion structure of the cheek pads is slightly reduced to slightly flattened (4). The cheeks are fully developed and the face is round.

4.4.3 Neck and chin

The structure of the neck and chin is assessed by four indicators. Indicator 4. The neck and chin overlap, the fat is doubled or tripled and closes the neck. Indicator 3.

Body Length (CM)	Body Weight (Kg)						
	-3 SD	-2 SD	-1SD	Median	+1SD	+2 SD	+3 SD
45.0	1.9	2.1	2.3	2.5	2.7	3.0	3.3
45.5	2.0	2.1	2.3	2.5	2.8	3.1	3.4
46.0	2.0	2.2	2.4	2.6	2.9	3.2	3.5
46.5	2.1	2.3	2.5	2.7	3.0	3.3	3.6
47.0	2.2	2.4	2.6	2.8	3.1	3.4	3.7
47.5	2.2	2.4	2.6	2.9	3.2	3.5	3.8
48.0	2.3	2.5	2.7	3,0	3.3	3.6	4.0
48.5	2.4	2.6	2.8	3.1	3.4	3.7	4.1
49.0	2.4	2.6	2.9	3.2	3.5	3.8	4.2
49.5	2.5	2.7	3.0	3.3	3.6	3.9	4.3
50.0	2.6	2.8	3.1	3.4	3.7	4.0	4.5
50.5	2.7	2.9	3.2	3.5	3.8	4.2	4.6
51.0	2.8	3.0	3.3	3.6	3.9	4.3	4.8
51.5	2.8	3.1	3.4	3.7	4.0	4.4	4.9
52.0	2.9	3.2	3.5	3.8	4.2	4.6	5.1
52.5	3.0	3.3	3.6	3.9	4.3	4.7	5.2
53.0	3.1	3.4	3.7	4.0	4.4	4.9	5.4
53.5	3.2	3.5	3.8	4.2	4.6	5.0	5.5
54.0	3.3	3.6	3.9	4.3	4.7	5.2	5.7
54.5	3.4	3.7	4.0	4.4	4.8	5.3	5.9
55.0	3.5	3.8	4.2	4.5	5.0	5.5	6.1
55.5	3.6	3.9	4.3	4.7	5.1	5.7	6.3
56.0	3.7	4.0	4.4	4.8	5.3	5.8	6.4
56.5	3.8	4.1	4.5	5.0	5.4	6.0	6.6
57.0	3.9	4.3	4.6	5.1	5.6	6.1	6.8
57.5	4.0	4.4	4.8	5.2	5.7	6.3	7.0
58.0	4.1	4.5	4.9	5.4	5.9	6.4	7.1
58.5	4.2	4.6	5.0	5.5	6.0	6.6	7.3
59.0	4.3	4.7	5.1	5.6	6.2	6.8	7.5
59.5	4.4	4.8	5.3	5.7	6.3	6.9	7.7
60.0	4.5	4.9	5.4	5.9	6.4	7.1	7.8
60.5	4.6	5.0	5.5	6.0	6.6	7.3	8.0
61.0	4.7	5.1	5.6	6.1	6.7	7.4	8.2
61.5	4.8	5.2	5.7	6.3	6.9	7.6	8.4
62.0	4.9	5.3	5.8	6.4	7.0	7.7	8.5
62.5	5.0	5.4	5.9	6.5	7.1	7.8	8.7
63.0	5.1	5.5	6.0	6.6	7.3	8.0	8.8
63.5	5.2	5.6	6.2	6.7	7.4	8.1	9.0

64.0	5.3	5.7	6.3	6.9	7.5	8.3	9.1
64.5	5.4	5.8	6.4	7.0	7.6	8.4	9.3
65.0	5.5	5.9	6.5	7.1	7.8	8.6	9.5
65.5	5.5	6.0	6.6	7.2	7.9	8.7	9.6
66.0	5.6	6.1	6.7	7.3	8.0	8.8	9.8
66.5	5.7	6.2	6.8	7.4	8.1	9.0	9.9
67.0	5.8	6.3	6.9	7.5	8.3	9.1	10.0
67.5	5.9	6.4	7.0	7.6	8.4	9.2	10.2
68.0	6.0	6.5	7.1	7.7	8.5	9.4	10.3
68.5	6.1	6.6	7.2	7.9	8.6	9,5	10.5
69.0	6.1	6.7	7.3	8.0	8.7	9.6	10.6
69.5	6.2	6.8	74	8.1	8.8	9.7	10.7
70.0	6.3	69	7.5	8.2	9.0	9.9	10.9

This table describes the standard weight according to body length (weight/ height) based on the threshold (Z-Score) for girls to be declared: severely wasted (< -3 SD), wasted (-3 SD to > -2 SD), good nutrition (-2SD to +1SD), possible risk of overweight (> +1 SD to +2SD), Obese (>+3SD).

Table 3.
Standard weight-for-height z score girls aged ***Tables*** *2 and 3 [22].*

The fat on the neck is slightly reduced, and the fat on the chin is thin. Indicator 2. Thin chin fat pad, visible neck. Indicator 1. No fat folds on the chin and neck look loose, and very clearly visible. Wrinkle skin.

4.4.4 Arm

The structure of the arm is assessed by four indicators. Indicator 4. Fully rounded sleeves, absent accordion pleats. Indicator 3. The arm has a little fat, there are folds of skin in the elbow or triceps area. Indicator 2 Small arms to the accordion. Indicator 1 The forearms have very thin skin, and loose skin and are easy to grip and pull from the elbow.

4.4.5 Foot

Measurements are the same as for the arm.

4.4.6 Behind the scapula

The rear structure is rated on four indicators. Indicator 4, the skin in the interscapular area is difficult to pull. Indicator 3. Slightly retractable skin Indicator 2. Skin is loose and easy to pull. Indicator 1 no fat, wrinkled skin and loose skin, easy to pull.

4.4.7 Buttocks

The rear structure is assessed based on four indicators. Indicator 4 gluteal fat pads are round and full. Indicator 3. looks a bit fat. Indicator 2. Significantly reduces fat and wrinkles. In indicator 1 there is almost no gluteal fat and the skin of the upper posterior buttock is loose and very wrinkled.

4.4.8 Chest

The structure of the chest is assessed by four indicators. Indicator 4. Chest full, rounded, ribs not visible. Indicator 3 intercostal spaces are slightly visible. The

Age (Month)	Height/Length Body						
	-3 SD	-2 SD	-1SD	Median	+1SD	+2 SD	+3 SD
0	44.2	46,1	48	49.9	51.8	53.7	55.6
1	48.9	50.8	52.8	54.7	56.7	58.6	60.6
2	52.4	54.4	56.4	58.4	60.4	62.4	64.4
3	55.3	57.3	59.4	61.4	63.5	65.5	67.6
4	57.6	59.7	61.8	63.9	66.0	68.0	79.1
5	59.6	61.7	63.8	65.9	68.0	70.1	72.2
6	61.2	63.3	65.5	67.6	69.8	71.9	74.0
7	62.7	64.8	67.0	69.2	71.3	73.5	75.7
8	64.0	66.2	68.4	70.6	72.8	75.0	77.2
9	65.2	67.5	69.7	72.0	74.2	76.5	78.7
10	66.4	68.7	71.0	73.3	75.6	77.9	80.1
11	67.6	69.9	72.2	74.5	76.9	79.2	81.5
12	68.6	71.0	73.4	75.7	78.1	80.5	82.9
13	69.6	72.1	74.5	76.9	79.3	81.8	84.2
14	70.6	73.1	75.6	78.0	80.5	83.0	85.5
15	71.6	74.1	76.6	79.1	81.7	84.2	86.7
16	72.5	75.0	77.6	80.2	82.8	85.4	88.0
17	73.3	76.0	78.6	81.2	83.9	86.5	89.2
18	74.2	76.9	79.6	82.3	85.0	87.7	90.4
19	75.0	77.7	80.5	83.2	86.0	88.8	91.5
20	75.8	78.6	81.4	84.2	87.0	89.8	92.6
21	76.5	79.4	82.3	85.1	88.0	90.9	93.8
22	77.2	80.2	84.1	86.0	89.0	91.9	94.9
23	78.0	81.0	83.9	86.9	89.9	92.9	95.9
24*	78.7	81.7	84.8	87.8	90.9	93.9	97.0

**Weight measurement is done with the child on his back [22].*
This table describe body length according to age with in boys with criteria: severely stunted (< -3 SD), stunted (-3 SD to <-2 SD), Normal (-2 SD to +3 SD), tall (> +3 SD).

Table 4.
Standard Height/Length for age z score (HAZ) aged boys 0-24 month.

Age (Month)	Height/Length Body						
	-3 SD	-2 SD	-1SD	Median	+1SD	+2 SD	+3 SD
0	43.6	45.4	47.3	49.1	51.0	52.9	54.7
1	47.8	49.8	51.7	53.7	55.7	57.6	59.5
2	51.0	53.0	55.0	57.1	59.1	61.1	63.2
3	53.5	55.6	57.7	59.8	61.9	64.0	66.1
4	66.6	57.8	59.9	62.1	64.3	66.4	68.6
5	57.4	59.6	61.8	64.0	66.2	68.5	70.7
6	58.9	61.2	63.5	65.7	68.0	70.3	72.5
7	60.3	62.7	65.0	67.3	69.6	71.9	74.2
8	61.7	64.0	66.0	68.7	71.1	73.5	57.8
9	62.9	65.3	67.7	70.1	72.6	75.0	77.4
10	64.1	66.5	69.0	71.5	73.9	76.4	78.9
11	65.2	67.7	70.3	72.8	75.3	77.8	80.3
12	66.3	68.9	74.0	74.0	76.6	79.2	81.7
13	67.3	70.0	72.6	75.2	77.8	80.5	83.1
14	68.3	71.0	73.7	76.4	79.1	81.7	84.4
15	69.3	72.0	74.8	77.5	80.2	83.0	85.7
16	70.2	73.0	75.8	78.5	81.4	84.2	87.0
17	71.1	74.0	76.8	79,7	82.5	86.4	88.2
18	72.0	74.9	77.8	80.7	83.6	86.5	89.4
19	72.8	75.8	78.8	81.7	84.7	87.6	90.6
20	73.7	76.7	79.7	82.7	85.7	88.7	91.7
21	74.5	77.5	80.6	83.7	86.7	89.8	92.9
22	75.2	78.4	81.5	84.6	87.7	90.8	94.0
23	76.0	79.2	82.3	85.5	88.7	91.9	95.0
24*	76.7	80.0	83.2	86.4	89.6	92.9	96.1

** Weight measurement is done with the child on his back [22].*
This table describes body length according to age in girls with criteria: severely stunted (< -3 SD), stunted (-3 SD to <-2 SD), Normal (-2 SD to +3 SD), tall (> +3 SD).

Table 5.
Standard Height/Length for age z score (HAZ) aged girls 0-24 month.

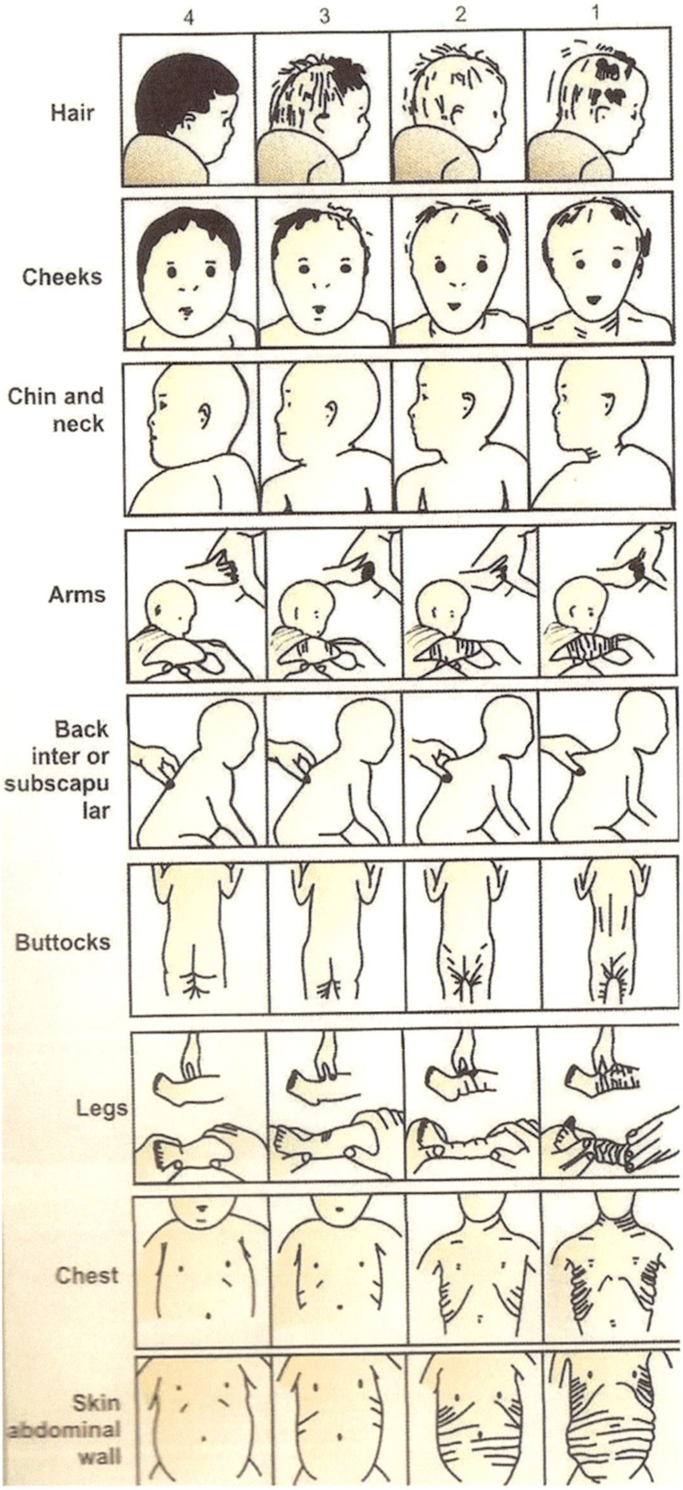

Figure 2.
Nutrition assessment with CAN Score [21].

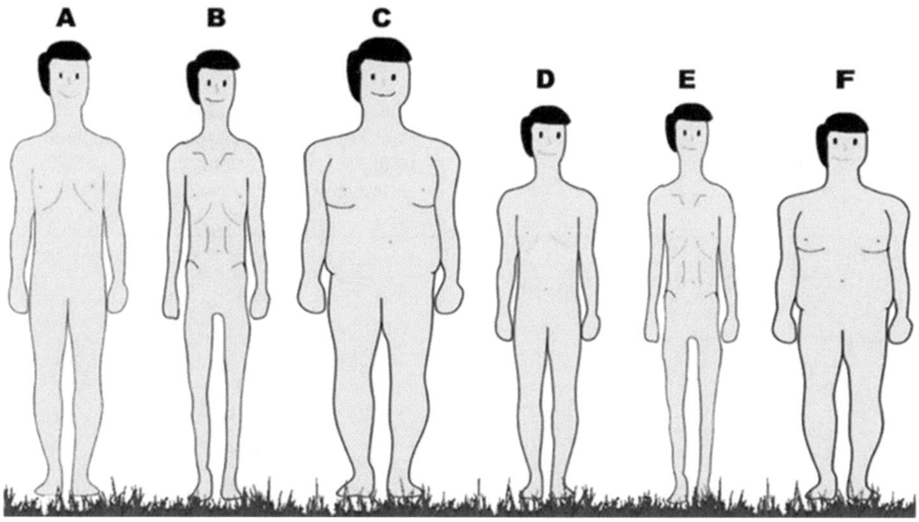

Figure 3.
Anthropometric classification of nutritional status (adapted to the Waterlow classification) of children under five [21].

Project	CANSCORE			
	4	3	2	1 point
Hair	Thick, dense, smooth, satin-tike, easy to comb	Thick, Scarce, there is little hair straight	Hair thin, straight and put up with more hair	Sparse, straight and erect hair, the hair bundle associated with reduced pigmentation
Cheek	Plump, round face	Slightly reduced fat	Significantly reduced	Fat is almost gone, narrow face
Neck chin	Fat overlap into double or triple chin, neck cover	Slightly reduced fat chin, the neck can be seen	Fat pad thin chin, neck revealed	Chin fat disappears, the neck is clear, loose skin, wrinkle
Arm	Fullness, can not lift the skin	Arm a little thin, check on the pressure of hands, the accordion-like folds can be formed	Small arms, to form accordion-like folds	Very little fat, loose skin, accordion-like folds significantly
Back	Inter-scapular area of skin can not be picked	Little to lift the skin	Easy to lift and skin	Loose skin, easy to lift, wrinkles can form
Buttock	Fat pad thickness	Slightly reduced fat	Significantly reduced fat, hips tip, wrinkle	Fat disappears, fight wrinkles, loose skin and a very, kind of hip, such as pipe
Leg	Described with the same arm	Described with the same arm	Described with the same arm	Described with the same arm
Chest	Full, see the intercostal space	Intercostal space slightly visible	Intercostal space revealed	Intercostal space very dear, obvious loss of subcutaneous tissue

Project	CANSCORE			
	4	3	2	1 point
Abdomen	Fullness, thickness of subcutaneous fat	Slightly reduced fat	Abdominal wall thinning, can form the accordion-like folds	Abdominal bulging or boat-shaped abdomen, loose skin, can form the accordion-like folds

Source: [21].

Table 6.
Can scoring.

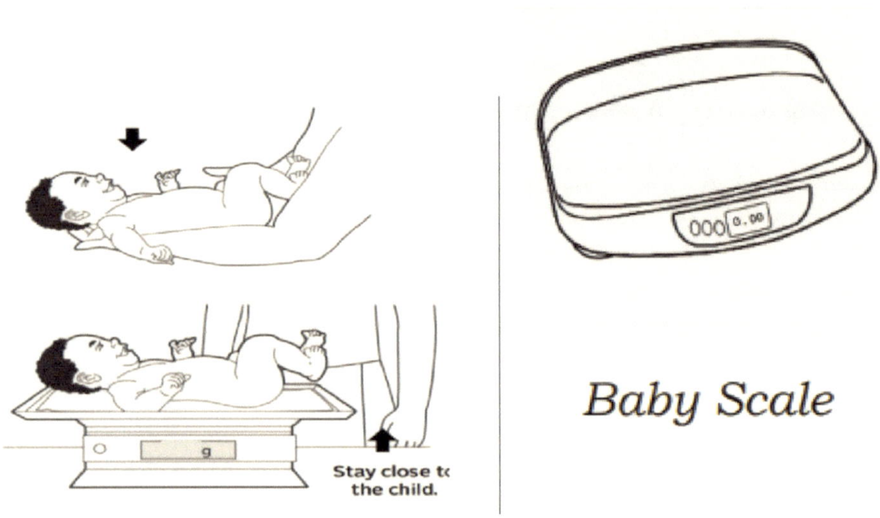

Figure 4.
Weight baby scales [22].

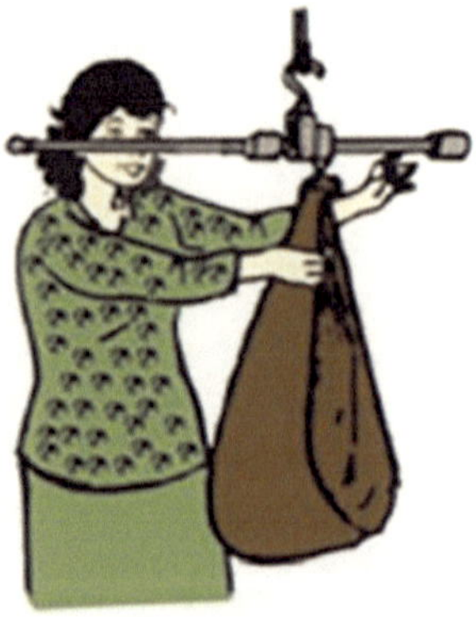

Figure 5.
Dacin tripod scale. This scale used to assess the weight of babies under five years old. This scale uses cloth material that can be folded and is easy to carry. This scale is usually used in posyandu services [22].

indicators of the 2 intercostal spaces are visible. Indicator 1; the ribs are increasingly prominent with loss of intercostal tissue.

4.4.9 Abdomen

The abdominal structure is assessed in four categories. Indicator 4. Skin is full, rounded, and not sagging. Indicator 3 reduces fat. Indicator 2 is thinning of the

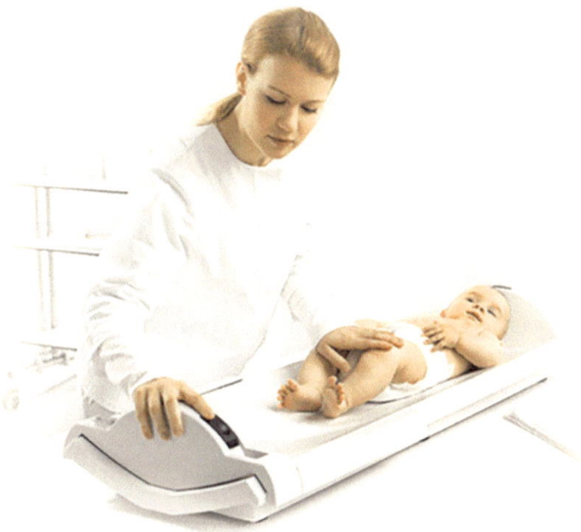

Figure 6.
Infantometer scale for body height. Measuring tools used by Indonesia in health services at Community Health Centers and Hospitals. The tool measures the baby's height from head to toe [22].

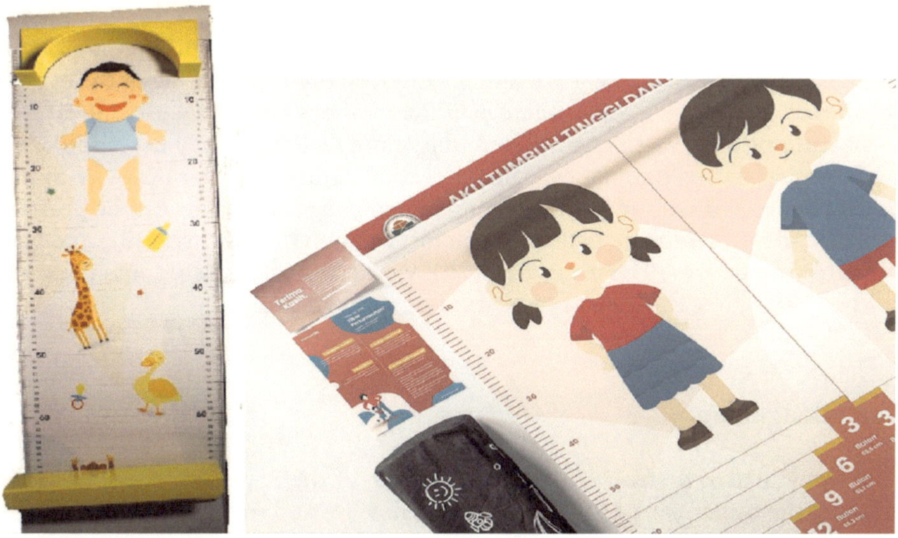

Figure 7.
Growth Mat scale. Growth Mat is a height measuring instrument made of wood and plastic. This tool is still used in Indonesia in Posyandu services. The tool is foldable and easy to carry [22].

abdominal wall from accordion to crease. Indicator 1 belly or scaphoid, but with very loose skin, easy to remove.

Nutritional status based on the cut of point CANScore divided by two that is score ≥ 25 They stated that the baby has good nutrition, and score < 25 declared as a child with undernutrition (**Figures 2** and **3**) [21]. Measurement instruments CAN Score can be seen in **Table 6**.

4.5 Measuring tools for detecting stunting, wasting in children

4.5.1 Weight scales

Infantometer: Measuring baby's weight (baby scale) (**Figure 4**).

Weighing gloves are used in posyandu throughout Indonesia. An instrument used to measure body weight (**Figure** 5).

4.5.2 Height scale

Infantometer: a measuring tool from abroad that is used for babies and toddlers (**Figure 6**).

4.5.3 Growth mat

Growth mat is a stunting early detection tool used in posyandu throughout Indonesia. This tool is used to measure the body length of children under the age of two (**Figure** 7).

5. Conclusions

Stunting and wasting are characteristic features of neonatal and infant growth disorders. Stunting and wasting are influenced by many factors. One of the events is a problem that occurs since the neonate is in the mother's womb. One of the efforts to prevent stunting and wasting from becoming more serious is early detection of the risk of stunting during pregnancy. Then detection continued after birth. With the hope that the risk of stunting, and wasting in neonates and infants can be prevented. This book can be a reference to help obtain information to detect stunting and wasting in neonates and infants. The users are health workers, health cadres, and the community who help reduce the incidence of stunting and wasting.

Acknowledgements

We would like to thank the Ministry of Health of the Republic of Indonesia for facilitating the use of baby growth measuring devices and socializing research on maternal and infant health and stunting. To the Jakarta 1 Health Polytechnic for promoting research on maternal and infant health and stunting.

Conflict of interest

There is no conflict of interest in writing a chapter book.

Acronyms and abbreviations

COVID-19	Coronavirus disease 2019
WHZ	Weight-for-height Z-scores
HAZ	Height-for-age z-score
IMD	Inisiasi menyusi dini/early initiation of breastfeeding
ANC	Ante natal care
WB/BL or WB/HB	Weight/Body or Weight Body/Hight Body
CAN	Clinical nutritional assessment

Author details

Suryani Manurung
Health Polytechnic Jakarta 1, Ministry of Health, Jakarta, Indonesia

*Address all correspondence to: suryanimanurung19@gmail.com

References

[1] National Institute of Health Research and Development of The Indonesia Ministry of Health. Indonesia Basic Health Survey (Riskesdas): The 2018. Jakarta: National Institute of Health Research and Development of The Indonesia Ministry of Health. Available from: http://labmandat.litbang.depkes.go.id/images/download/laporan/RKD/2018/Laporan%7B%5C_%7DNasional%7B%5C_%7DRKD2018%7B%5C_%7DFINAL.pd; 2018 [Accessed: December 1, 2023]

[2] The Ministry of Health of The Republic of Indonesia. Report on the Implementation of the March 2019 Susenas Integration and the 2019 Indonesian Toddler Nutritional Status Survey. Jakarta: The Ministry of Health of The Republic of Indonesia; 2019. Available from: https://cegahstunting.id/unduhan/publikasi-data/

[3] UNICEF. Indonesia: Number of Malnourished Children Could Increase Sharply Due to COVID-19 unless Swift Action Is Taken. Jakarta: UNICEF; 2020. pp. 1-3. Available from: https://www.unicef.org/indonesia/press-releases/number-of-malnourished-children-in-indonesia-could-increase-sharply-due-to-covid-19

[4] Titaley CR, Ariawan I, Hapsari D, et al. Determinants of the stunting of children in Indonesia: A multilevel analysis of the 2013 Indonesia basic health survey. Nutrients. 2019;**11**:1160. Available from: https://www.mdpi.com/2072-6643/11/5/1106

[5] Saleh A, Syahrul S, Hadju V, et al. Role of maternal in preventing stunting: A systematic review. Gaceta Sanitaria. 2021;**35**:S576-S582

[6] Soliman A, De SV, Alaaraj N, et al. Early and long term consequences of nutritional stunting: From childhood to adulthood. Acta Bio-Medica. 2021;**9**:1-12. Available from: https://www.ncbi.nlm.nih.gov/pmc/articles/PMC7975963/

[7] Prendergast AJ, Humphrey JH. The stunting syndrome in developing countries. Paediatrics and International Child Health. 2014;**34**:250-265. Available from: https://www.ncbi.nlm.nih.gov/pmc/articles/PMC4232245/

[8] UNICEF/WHO/Word Bank Group. Level and Trends in Child Malnutrition. New York: UNICEF; 2023. pp. 1-9. Available from: https://data.unicef.org/resources/jme-report-2023/

[9] Sartika AN, Khoirunnisa M, Meiyetriani E, et al. Prenatal and postnatal stunting at age 0-11 months: Across sectional study Indonesia. PLoS One. 2021;**16**:1-14. Available from: https://journals.plos.org/plosone/article?id=10.1371/journal.pone.0254662

[10] Lukman TNE, Anwar F, Riyadi H, et al. Birth weight and length associated with stunting among children under-five in Indonesia. Jurnal Gizi dan Pangan. 2021;**16**:99-108

[11] Laksono AD, Wulandari RD, Amaliah N, et al. Stunting among children under two years in Indonesia: Does maternal education matter? PLoS One. 2022;**17**:1-11. Available from: https://journals.plos.org/plosone/article?id=10.1371/journal.pone.0271509

[12] Gale CR, O'Callaghan FJ, Godfrey KM, et al. Critical periods of brain growth and cognitive function in children. Brain. 2004;**127**:321-329. Available from: https://pubmed.ncbi.nlm.nih.gov/14645144/

[13] Walker SP, Wachs TD, Gardner JM, et al. Child development: Risk factors for adverse outcomes in developing countries. Lancet. 2007;**369**:145-157. Available from: https://www.thelancet.com/journals/lancet/article/PIIS0140-6736(07)60076-2/fulltext

[14] Pham BN, Silas VD, Okely AD, et al. Measuring wasting and stunting prevalence among children under years of Ag and associated risk factors ini Papua New Guinea: New evidance from the comprehensive health and epidemiological surveillance system. Frontiers in Nutrition. 2021;**8**:1-13. Available from: https://www.frontiersin.org/articles/10.3389/fnut.2021.622660/full

[15] Sari DR, Fatmaningrum W, Suryawan A. Hubungan etnis, ASI ekslusif dan berat badan lahir dengan stunting pada balita usia 11-59 bulan di Surabaya. Indonesian Midwifery and Health Sciences Journal. 2019;**3**:320-330. Available from: https://e-journal.unair.ac.id/index.php/IMHSJ

[16] Suratri MAL, Putro G, Rachmat B, et al. Risk factors for stunting among children under five years. International Journal of Environmental Research and Public Health. 2023;**20**:1-13. DOI: 10.3390/ijerph20021640

[17] WHO. Physical Status: The Use and Interpretation of Antropometri. Geneva: WHO Library; 1995. Available from: https://apps.who.int/iris/bitstream/handle/10665/37003/WHO_TRS_854.pdf?sequence=1&isAllowed=y

[18] Gonete AT, Kassahun B, Mekonnen EG, et al. Stunting at birth and associated factors among newborns delivered at the University of Gondar Comprehensive Specialized Referral Hospital. PLoS One. 2021;**16**:e0245528. DOI: 10.1371/journal.pone.0245528

[19] Chhabra P, Gupta A, Thakur N. Complementary feeding practices and nutritional status of children (6–23 months) in an urban resettlement colony of East Delhi. Indian Journal of Community Medicine. 2021;**46**:528-532. Available from: https://www.ncbi.nlm.nih.gov/pmc/articles/PMC8575192/

[20] Desyanti C, Nindya TS. Hubungan riwayat penyakit diare dan praktik higiene dengan kejadian stunting pada balita usia 24-59 bulan di wilayah Kerja Puskesmas Simolawang, Surabaya. Open Access Under. 2017;**1**:243-251

[21] da Ferreira HS. Anthropometric assessment of children's nutritional status: A new approach based on an adaptation of Waterlow's classification. BMC Pediatrics. 2020;**20**:1-11. Available from: https://link.springer.com/content/pdf/10.1186/s12887-020-1940-6.pdf

[22] Kementerian Kesehatan Republik Indonesia. In: Dan AD, editor. Standard antropometri penilaian satatus gizi anak. pertama ed. Jakarta: Kemenkes RI; 2011. Available from: https://med.unhas.ac.id/kedokteran/wp-content/uploads/2017/03/buku-sk-antropometri-2010-1.pdf

Chapter 5

Vaginal Seeding in Term Cesarean Section Is a Mandatory Condition for Improvement of Neonatal Health

Panagiotis Tsikouras, Xanthi Anthoulaki, Efthimios Oikonomou, Anastasia Bothou, Konstantinos Nikolettos, Alexios Alexiou, Dimitrios Kyriakou, Theopi Nalbanti, Sonia Kotanidou, Nektaria Kritsotaki, Natalia Sahnova, Aise Chatzi Ismail, Vlasios Spanakis, Georgios Iatrakis and Nikolaos Nikolettos

Abstract

The human vaginal microbiota is an important component of the defense system to fight microbial and viral infections. During pregnancy, a significant decrease in overall diversity is observed in the vaginal flora, and there is an increase in stability as the composition of the vaginal flora changes gradually. These alterations are linked to a decrease in vaginal pH and an augmentation in vaginal secretions. The composition of the vaginal microbiome changes according to gestational age, with its composition in advanced weeks of pregnancy resembling that of nonpregnant women. There is supporting evidence for the existence of differences in the neonate's microbiome between those born *via* C-section and those delivered vaginally. The evidence suggests that this difference is a result of the changes that occur in the mother's microbiome, particularly in the vagina. The vaginal microbiome serves as a crucial barrier between the external environment and the intra-amniotic cavity. The vaginal microbiome appears to play a significant role as an additional defense mechanism of the mother and, consequently, the fetus. Any abnormalities in this microbiome can potentially impact the pregnancy and perinatal outcome.

Keywords: term pregnancies, cesarean section, vaginal delivery vaginal seeding, elective cesarean section with vaginal seeding, perinatal outcome

1. Introduction

Until the beginning of the twentieth century, it was believed that the fetus came into the world free of microbes. Today, there are numerous indications that disprove this hypothesis and suggest that there is already a presence of microbes in the fetal-placental unit. A useful model for examining the causes of numerous disorders and the development of human health is the neonatal microbiome. Multiple studies have described the importance of the first 1000 days of life when basic physiological exposures to microbes can have profound effects on future health. The establishment of a healthy microbiome, comprising trillions of microbial cells and their respective genomes, is critical during this period [1–3]. The neonatal microbiome begins as early as the prenatal period, where many studies suggest that the maternal microbiota colonizes the infant through the *in utero* environment. From here, mode of delivery, breastfeeding, diet, and environment lead to a rapid expansion of bacterial complexity as the microbiome becomes established. This stable trajectory of progressive bacterial colonization becomes critical for immune priming, normal function in multiple organ systems, and lays the foundation for future health. The mode of delivery, whether by cesarean section or vaginal delivery, can influence the neonatal immune system and subsequent susceptibility to infections. Identifying vaginal infections that are dangerous to pregnancy and the fetus from those that are bothersome but harmless and manageable, as well as their precise management, is a challenge for medical experts [4, 5].

The following chapter is the result of a literature review in order to investigate the effects of vaginitis on pregnancy outcomes. This refers to an investigation of the normal microflora of the vagina, its defense mechanisms, and the microorganisms that colonize it. The second part refers to the pathological colonizations of the vagina, the types of vaginitis that cause them, and their diagnosis. Next, the changes that the vagina undergoes during pregnancy, its pathology from the colonization of pathogenic microorganisms, and their treatment are described. Finally, the effects of vaginitis on the outcome of pregnancy are described, with pathologies such as chorioamnionitis, premature birth, and spontaneous abortion.

1.1 Background and context

In recent years, vaginal seeding has drawn interest as a potential strategy to improve the development of the neonatal microbiome. The community of microbes that live in the human body, notably the gut, skin, and mucous membranes, is referred to as the microbiome. It is essential for the development of the immune system, metabolism, and defense against pathogens, among other elements of health. The newborn is exposed to a wide variety of germs in the birth canal during a vaginal birth. This exposure is believed to contribute to the initial colonization of the infant's gut with beneficial bacteria, such as Bifidobacterium and Lactobacillus species. These bacteria are associated with immune system development, regulation of inflammation, and protection against certain diseases.

Cesarean section (C-section) delivery, however, bypasses the vaginal birth canal, resulting in a different microbial exposure for the newborn. Infants born *via* C-section tend to have a microbiome composition that differs from those born vaginally. Research has shown that these differences may have implications for the infant's health as C-section-born infants have been found to have an increased risk of certain health conditions, such as allergies, asthma, atopic disease, obesity, and autoimmune disorders [3–5].

Vaginal seeding is proposed as a method to mimic the microbial exposure of a vaginal birth for infants born *via* C-section. It involves the collection of maternal vaginal fluids, typically using a sterile swab, which is then transferred onto the newborn's skin or mouth within the first moments after birth. The goal is to introduce the mother's vaginal microbiota to the newborn, potentially promoting a microbial colonization pattern similar to that of a vaginal birth. Vaginal seeding is still a contentious issue, despite the fact that it has attracted interest as a potential strategy to affect the newborn microbiota. The possibility for hazardous microbes, such as pathogens and bacteria, resistant to antibiotics, to be transmitted from the mother to the newborn has given rise to safety concerns. The lack of standardized protocols for evaluating the maternal vaginal microbiota and screening for infections poses challenges for implementing this practice. Given the potential impact of the neonatal microbiome on health outcomes and the increasing rates of C-section deliveries, there is a need to better understand the potential benefits and risks associated with vaginal seeding. Ongoing research aims to investigate its effects on the neonatal microbiome composition, immune development, and long-term health outcomes. The findings of these studies have the potential to inform clinical practice, guidelines, and decision-making regarding vaginal seeding [3–7].

1.2 Rationale for studying vaginal seeding

The rationale for studying vaginal seeding lies in the growing interest in understanding the potential impact of this practice on neonatal health outcomes. As the rates of cesarean section deliveries continue to rise globally, there is a need to explore interventions that could mitigate the potential differences in microbial exposure and associated health risks between infants born *via* C-section and those born vaginally [3–7].

1. Enhancement of neonatal microbiome: The neonatal microbiome plays a crucial role in immune development, metabolic processes, and overall health. Vaginal seeding is proposed as a method to introduce the maternal vaginal microbiota to infants born *via* C-section, potentially enhancing the establishment of a more diverse and balanced microbiome. By replicating the microbial exposure of a vaginal birth, vaginal seeding aims to promote the colonization of beneficial bacteria, which may contribute to optimal immune development and reduce the risk of certain health conditions.

2. Potential health benefits: Several studies and anecdotal reports have suggested potential benefits associated with vaginal seeding. These include a reduced risk of allergies, asthma, autoimmune disorders, and metabolic conditions, such as obesity. Exploring the efficacy of vaginal seeding in influencing these health outcomes could provide valuable insights into preventive measures and interventions to optimize neonatal health.

3. Addressing health disparities: Studies have shown that infants born *via* C-section have a higher risk of certain health conditions compared to those born vaginally. By investigating the potential impact of vaginal seeding, researchers aim to address these health disparities and explore strategies to improve the health outcomes of infants born *via* C-section.

4. Clinical decision-making: The growing interest in vaginal seeding has led to varied practices and opinions among healthcare professionals. Conducting research on vaginal seeding can provide evidence-based guidance for healthcare providers, enabling them to make informed decisions and recommendations regarding this practice. Understanding the potential benefits and risks of vaginal seeding is essential for developing standardized protocols, identifying appropriate candidates, and ensuring safe implementation.

5. Ethical considerations: Vaginal seeding raises ethical considerations regarding safety, informed consent, and equitable access to the intervention. Investigating vaginal seeding helps to address these ethical concerns and inform discussions surrounding the risks and benefits of the practice, ensuring that healthcare decisions are made in the best interest of the newborns and their families.

In summary, studying vaginal seeding is important to explore its potential to enhance the neonatal microbiome, mitigate health risks associated with C-section deliveries, and improve neonatal health outcomes. By understanding the rationale behind vaginal seeding and conducting rigorous research, healthcare professionals can make informed decisions and provide evidence-based recommendations to optimize neonatal care [7–9].

2. Literature review

2.1 Overview of the neonatal microbiome and its importance in health

The neonatal microbiome refers to the collection of microorganisms, including bacteria, viruses, fungi, and other microbes, that inhabit the newborn's body, particularly the gut, skin, and mucous membranes. The newborn microbiome experiences rapid development and is essential for many aspects of development and health. During pregnancy, the fetus is believed to be in a relatively sterile environment. However, upon birth, the neonate is rapidly colonized by microorganisms from the surrounding environment, primarily influenced by the mode of delivery, feeding practices, maternal factors, and exposure to the external environment. The early establishment of a diverse and balanced neonatal microbiome is important for multiple physiological processes [7–9].

Immune system development: The neonatal microbiome plays a crucial role in the maturation and development of the immune system. The presence of beneficial bacteria in the gut stimulates the production of specific immune cells and regulatory molecules, promoting immune tolerance and preventing exaggerated immune responses. The interaction between the microbiome and the immune system is essential for the proper functioning of immune defense mechanisms and protection against infections [7–9].

Metabolic processes: The neonatal microbiome is involved in various metabolic processes, including the fermentation of dietary components and the production of essential metabolites. Beneficial bacteria in the gut can break down complex carbohydrates that are indigestible by the host, producing short-chain fatty acids and other metabolites that provide energy to the host cells and contribute to overall metabolic homeostasis [9–11].

Protection against pathogens: A defense against possible infections is provided by the newborn microbiota. Pathogens are kept from colonizing and overgrowing by beneficial bacteria in the gut and on the skin, which compete with them for nutrition and space. Additionally, they create antimicrobial chemicals that can obstruct the development of viruses and bacteria that cause disease [9–11].

Maturation of organ systems: The neonatal microbiome has been implicated in the maturation and development of various organ systems. It influences the development and integrity of the intestinal epithelial barrier, aiding in nutrient absorption and preventing the translocation of harmful substances into the bloodstream. Additionally, the microbiome can influence the development of the central nervous system and the modulation of neurotransmitters, potentially affecting neurodevelopmental processes.

Association with health and disease: Alterations in the neonatal microbiome have been associated with various health conditions and disease outcomes. Dysbiosis, an imbalance or disruption in the microbial composition, has been linked to an increased risk of allergies, asthma, obesity, autoimmune disorders, gastrointestinal disorders (such as necrotizing enterocolitis), and even neurodevelopmental disorders. Understanding the role of the neonatal microbiome in these health conditions can help develop targeted interventions and strategies for prevention and treatment [9–11].

The neonatal microbiome is a dynamic ecosystem that influences various aspects of health and development. Its establishment and composition in the early stages of life play a crucial role in immune system maturation, metabolic processes, pathogen defense, and the development of organ systems. Understanding the importance of the neonatal microbiome provides insights into the potential impact of interventions, such as vaginal seeding on health outcomes and underscores the need for further research to optimize neonatal health [9–11].

2.2 Exploration of factors influencing the neonatal microbiome, including mode of delivery

The composition and development of the neonatal microbiome are influenced by various factors, including the mode of delivery. Here, we explore the factors that impact the neonatal microbiome, with a specific focus on the influence of delivery mode.

2.2.1 Mode of delivery

Vaginal delivery: During a vaginal birth, the newborn is exposed to the microorganisms present in the birth canal, including bacteria from the maternal vaginal and fecal microbiota. This exposure leads to the colonization of the neonate's gut, skin, and mucosal surfaces with a diverse range of microorganisms, primarily bacteria. Infants born vaginally tend to have a microbiome composition characterized by an abundance of beneficial bacteria, such as Bifidobacterium and Lactobacillus species [9–11].

Cesarean section (C-section): Bypassing the birth canal, a C-section includes the surgical delivery of the infant through an incision in the belly and uterus. Infants delivered by C-section experience a different level of microbial exposure than those delivered vaginally. They are initially colonized by microorganisms present in the surrounding environment, including skin and hospital surfaces. The microbiome of C-section-born infants tends to be less diverse and dominated by bacteria associated with the hospital environment [11–13].

2.2.2 Maternal factors

Maternal microbiota: The composition of the maternal microbiota, particularly the vaginal and gut microbiota, can influence the initial colonization of the neonatal microbiome. The transfer of maternal microorganisms during vaginal birth contributes to the establishment of the neonatal microbiome. Differences in the maternal microbiota, such as bacterial diversity and composition, can impact the microbial transmission to the newborn.

Maternal health and lifestyle: Maternal health conditions, such as obesity, diabetes, and gestational infections, can influence the microbial composition and diversity transferred to the neonate. Maternal lifestyle factors, including diet, antibiotic use, and exposure to environmental factors, may also affect the microbiota and potentially impact the neonatal microbiome [11–13].

2.2.3 Breastfeeding

Breast milk composition: Prebiotics, other bioactive substances, and a wide variety of helpful bacteria are all present in breast milk, which helps some bacteria flourish in the neonatal gut. Lactobacillus and Bifidobacterium, two helpful bacteria that support the development of a healthy microbial community in the infant's gut, are found in breast milk.

Mode of feeding: Neonatal microbiota composition has been linked to breastfeeding vs. formula feeding. In order to encourage the construction of a healthy gut microbiome in the infant, breast milk helps to generate a more diversified and advantageous microbial community [11–13].

2.2.4 Environmental exposures

Early life exposures: Factors, such as the home environment, hygiene practices, and exposure to pets or siblings, can influence the neonatal microbiome. These early life exposures can introduce additional microorganisms and potentially impact the diversity and composition of the neonatal microbiome.

It makes it easier to understand the intricacies of microbial colonization throughout the early stages of life to be aware of the factors that affect the newborn microbiome such as the manner of delivery, maternal factors, nursing, and environmental exposures. It highlights how crucial it is to take these aspects into account when examining how interventions, such as vaginal seeding, affect the newborn microbiota and health consequences [11–13].

2.3 Introduction to vaginal seeding and its potential benefits and controversies

Vaginal seeding is an emerging practice that aims to mimic the microbial exposure of a vaginal birth for infants born *via* cesarean section (C-section). It involves transferring maternal vaginal fluids, including microorganisms, onto the newborn shortly after birth. The rationale behind vaginal seeding is to introduce beneficial bacteria from the mother's vaginal microbiota to the newborn, potentially influencing the establishment of the neonatal microbiome and promoting optimal immune development [13–17].

The potential benefits associated with vaginal seeding are rooted in the understanding that the early colonization of the neonatal gut with beneficial bacteria plays a crucial role in immune system maturation, metabolic processes, and protection against certain health conditions. Proponents of vaginal seeding hypothesize that by replicating the microbial exposure of a vaginal birth, this intervention may help restore the microbiome composition of C-section-born infants, making it more similar to that of vaginally delivered infants. This, in turn, could potentially lead to a reduced risk of certain health conditions such as allergies, asthma, obesity, and autoimmune disorders.

However, the practice of vaginal seeding is not without controversy and debates. One of the main concerns revolves around the potential transmission of harmful microorganisms from the maternal vaginal canal to the newborn. This includes the risk of transmitting pathogens such as group B Streptococcus, herpes simplex virus, or antibiotic-resistant bacteria. The lack of standardized protocols for evaluating the maternal vaginal microbiota and screening for infections poses challenges in ensuring the safety of vaginal seeding [13–17].

Additionally, the scientific evidence supporting the efficacy and safety of vaginal seeding is limited and often based on small-scale studies or anecdotal reports. The existing studies on vaginal seeding have reported conflicting findings, making it challenging to draw definitive conclusions. There is a need for larger, well-designed studies to evaluate the impact of vaginal seeding on the neonatal microbiome, immune development, and long-term health outcomes. Moreover, the practice of vaginal seeding is not currently recommended by major healthcare organizations, such as the American College of Obstetricians and Gynecologists (ACOG), due to safety concerns and the lack of sufficient evidence. In particular, the ACOG recommends that clinicians and patients avoid this practice, unless as part of an approved research protocol [13–18].

Addressing the controversies and debates surrounding vaginal seeding requires further research and scientific investigation. This includes developing standardized protocols for assessing the maternal vaginal microbiota, screening for infections, and evaluating the short- and long-term effects of vaginal seeding on neonatal health outcomes. The potential benefits and risks of vaginal seeding need to be carefully considered and weighed against each other with a focus on ensuring the safety and well-being of the newborns.

2.4 Review of existing literature on vaginal seeding, including studies on microbiome composition, immune development, and health outcomes

In recent years, several studies have investigated the impact of vaginal seeding on the neonatal microbiome composition, immune development, and various health outcomes. Here, we review the existing literature on vaginal seeding, highlighting key findings and insights in these areas.

Microbiome composition: Studies examining the neonatal microbiome composition following vaginal seeding have reported varying results. Some studies have shown that vaginal seeding leads to an increased abundance of bacteria associated with vaginal birth, such as Lactobacillus and Bifidobacterium species, in the gut and other body sites of C-section-born infants. These findings suggest that vaginal seeding can help establish a microbial community resembling that of infants born vaginally [19–23].

However, other studies have reported inconsistent or limited effects of vaginal seeding on the neonatal microbiome composition. Methodological differences, including variations in the timing and techniques of vaginal fluid transfer, sample collection methods, and analysis techniques, may contribute to the discrepancies in findings. Larger, well-controlled studies with standardized protocols are needed to further elucidate the impact of vaginal seeding on the neonatal microbiome composition [19–23].

Immune development: The influence of vaginal seeding on immune development in newborns has also been explored. Some studies have suggested that vaginal seeding may promote immune maturation such as indicated by changes in immune cell populations, cytokine profiles, and immune markers. These findings indicate that exposure to maternal vaginal microbiota through vaginal seeding may play a role in modulating immune responses and promoting immune tolerance.

However, the clinical significance and long-term implications of these immune changes remain unclear. Further, research is needed to establish a clear link between vaginal seeding and immune development, considering factors such as the timing and frequency of vaginal seeding, potential variations in immune outcomes, and the interplay with other factors influencing immune development [19–23].

Health outcomes: The potential impact of vaginal seeding on health outcomes in C-section-born infants has been a topic of interest. Some observational studies have reported associations between vaginal seeding and a reduced risk of certain health conditions, including allergies, asthma, and autoimmune disorders. These findings suggest that vaginal seeding may have long-term health benefits by influencing the neonatal microbiome and immune system [23–25].

However, the evidence on health outcomes and the clinical significance of these associations is limited and often based on small-scale studies or anecdotal reports. Larger, well-designed studies, including randomized controlled trials, are needed to further investigate the potential benefits and long-term effects of vaginal seeding on health outcomes. It is essential to consider potential confounding factors, such as breastfeeding practices and other early life exposures, when assessing the impact of vaginal seeding on health outcomes [23–27].

In summary, the existing literature on vaginal seeding indicates a potential influence on the neonatal microbiome composition, immune development, and health outcomes. While some studies suggest positive associations between vaginal seeding and beneficial outcomes, the evidence is limited, and conflicting results have been reported. Further, research, including larger-scale studies with standardized protocols, is necessary to establish a clearer understanding of the effects of vaginal seeding on the neonatal microbiome, immune development, and long-term health outcomes.

Despite the growing interest in vaginal seeding, there are several gaps in the current knowledge that need to be addressed through further research. These gaps include:

Lack of standardized protocols: There is a lack of standardized protocols for assessing the maternal vaginal microbiota, including methods for sample collection, processing, and analysis. Standardized protocols are crucial for ensuring consistency across studies and facilitating comparisons between different research findings [23–25].

Variations in vaginal seeding practices: Vaginal seeding practices vary widely across studies, including differences in the timing and techniques of vaginal fluid transfer, the selection of participants, and the criteria for determining eligibility. These variations make it difficult to draw definitive conclusions or compare results between studies. Standardized protocols for vaginal seeding are needed to establish consistency in practice and facilitate meaningful comparisons [25–29].

Small sample sizes: Many studies investigating vaginal seeding have relatively small sample sizes, which may limit the generalizability and statistical power of the findings. Larger-scale studies with adequate sample sizes are required to provide more robust evidence regarding the effects of vaginal seeding on the neonatal microbiome, immune development, and health outcomes.

Long-term follow-up studies: There are not enough long-term follow-up studies to evaluate the consequences of vaginal seeding after birth. Longitudinal studies that track infants exposed to vaginal seeding over an extended period are needed to evaluate the persistence of any observed effects and to assess potential health outcomes, including allergies, asthma, autoimmune disorders, and metabolic conditions.

Limited diversity of participants: Many studies on vaginal seeding have primarily focused on populations from developed countries, limiting the generalizability of the findings to other populations and settings. It is essential to include diverse populations, including those from different geographical regions and with varying sociocultural backgrounds, to understand the broader implications of vaginal seeding [25–29].

Safety concerns and screening protocols: Safety concerns regarding the potential transmission of harmful microorganisms during vaginal seeding need to be addressed. Standardized protocols for evaluating the maternal vaginal microbiota, including screening for infections and identification of potential pathogens, are necessary to ensure the safety of vaginal seeding procedures.

Mechanistic understanding: While studies have explored the effects of vaginal seeding on the neonatal microbiome and immune development, the underlying mechanisms are not well understood. Further, research is needed to elucidate the specific pathways through which vaginal seeding influences these processes and to identify the key microbial factors driving any observed effects. Addressing these gaps in the current knowledge will provide a more comprehensive understanding of vaginal seeding and its implications for neonatal health [29–31]. Large-scale, well-controlled studies with standardized protocols, long-term follow-up, diverse populations, and a focus on safety considerations are crucial for advancing our understanding of the potential benefits, risks, and mechanisms of action associated with vaginal seeding.

2.5 Consideration of the limitations of the included studies and potential sources of bias

It is important to acknowledge the limitations of the included studies and potential sources of bias as they can influence the interpretation and generalizability of the findings. Some common limitations and potential sources of bias in studies related to neonatal microbial colonization and mode of delivery include: (1). Sample size: Numerous research in this field can have sample sizes that are not very large, which could reduce the statistical power and generalizability of the findings. Small sample sizes might not accurately reflect the population's variety, which could result in selection bias. (2). Selection bias: Studies may recruit participants from specific populations or healthcare settings, leading to selection bias. This can affect the representativeness of the sample and limit the ability to extrapolate the findings to a broader population. (3). Retrospective design: Some studies may use retrospective designs, relying on medical records or previously collected data. Retrospective studies may suffer from incomplete or inaccurate data, and researchers may have limited control over the variables studied. (4). Confounding factors: The association between the technique of delivery and neonatal microbial colonization can be influenced by a number of confounding variables. These elements include nursing habits, gestational age, antibiotic use, maternal microbiome, and mother health. The results may be skewed if these factors are not properly taken into account. (5). Lack of standardization: The methods used to assess microbial colonization can vary between studies, making it challenging to compare results directly. Differences in sampling techniques, DNA extraction, sequencing methods, and data analysis may contribute to variability in findings. (6). Cross-sectional nature: Some studies may have a cross-sectional design, which captures data at a single time point. This design may not allow for the evaluation of changes in microbial colonization over time, limiting the understanding of the dynamics of neonatal microbiota. (7). Lack of long-term follow-up: Long-term follow-up of neonates beyond the immediate postnatal period is essential to assess the potential impact of early-life microbial colonization on later health outcomes. However, many studies may lack long-term follow-up data. (8). Vaginal seeding practice: Studies investigating the impact of vaginal seeding on neonatal microbial colonization are relatively new and may have limited data on the safety and long-term effects of this practice. This area requires further research to establish its clinical efficacy and safety. (9). Publication bias: Published studies may be more likely to report positive or statistically significant results, leading to publication bias. Negative or nonsignificant findings may be underreported, potentially skewing the overall literature on the topic. (10). To mitigate these limitations and potential sources of bias, future studies should aim for larger sample sizes, prospective designs, standardized methods, and rigorous control of confounding factors [31–33]. Additionally, conducting long-term follow-up studies can provide valuable insights into the lasting effects of neonatal microbial colonization on health outcomes. Collaborative efforts and multicenter studies can also enhance the generalizability of the findings and improve our understanding of the complex interactions between mode of delivery, neonatal microbial colonization, and health.

2.6 Addressing the controversies and debates surrounding vaginal seeding

Vaginal seeding is a controversial practice that involves exposing infants born *via* cesarean section to the maternal vaginal microbes shortly after birth. While some proponents of vaginal seeding suggest that it may help promote a more diverse and beneficial microbial colonization in cesarean-born infants, there are significant controversies and debates surrounding its safety, efficacy, and potential risks. Limited Scientific One of the main controversies surrounding vaginal seeding is the lack of robust scientific evidence supporting its safety and long-term benefits. Most studies on the topic have been small, and there is a need for larger, well-designed clinical trials to establish the safety and effectiveness of vaginal seeding. Introducing maternal vaginal microbes to cesarean-born infants carries the risk of transferring harmful bacteria or infections to the newborn. The vaginal microbiome is diverse, and it can include potentially pathogenic microorganisms that may pose health risks to the vulnerable newborns. Vaginal seeding is not a standardized medical procedure, and there is no consensus on the best method for performing it. Different practitioners may use varied techniques, which can lead to inconsistencies and potential risks. While the intent of vaginal seeding is to promote a more diverse and beneficial microbial colonization, there is a concern that it may lead to unintended consequences [33–39]. The introduction of foreign microbes could potentially disrupt the delicate balance of the infant's microbiome and have unknown effects on their health. Vaginal seeding raises ethical concerns as it involves exposing infants to a practice that has not been thoroughly studied for its safety and effectiveness. Inclusion in clinical trials may be complicated due to the need for informed consent and potential risks. Before considering vaginal seeding, the potential benefits must be carefully weighed against the potential risks. Cesarean section is a lifesaving procedure in many cases, and the risks associated with vaginal seeding must be justified by significant potential benefits. Some researchers suggest that breastfeeding and skin-to-skin contact may provide beneficial microbial exposure for cesarean-born infants without the risks associated with vaginal seeding [37–43]. More research is needed to explore alternative approaches to promote a healthy microbiome in cesarean-born infants. In conclusion, while vaginal seeding has gained attention as a potential method to influence neonatal microbial colonization, it remains a controversial and debated practice. The lack of substantial scientific evidence, potential infection risks, and ethical considerations warrant caution and careful consideration before adopting vaginal seeding as a standard practice. Further, research is needed to better understand the safety and long-term effects of vaginal seeding and to explore alternative strategies to promote a healthy microbial colonization in cesarean-born infants. Until then, it is essential for healthcare providers and parents to engage in informed discussions about the potential risks and benefits of vaginal seeding and make decisions based on the best available evidence and individual circumstances [43–49].

2.7 Suggestions for future research and recommendations for clinical practice

Future research in the field of neonatal microbial colonization and mode of delivery should focus on addressing the existing gaps in knowledge and providing more robust evidence to guide clinical practice. Here are some suggestions for future research and recommendations for clinical practice:

2.7.1 Future research

1. Long-term follow-up: Conduct longitudinal studies with long-term follow-up to understand the lasting effects of neonatal microbial colonization on health outcomes. This will help establish the association between early-life microbial exposure and the development of various health conditions later in life.

2. Randomized controlled trials: To assess the security and effectiveness of vaginal seeding, conduct sizable, and randomized controlled studies. In order to give trustworthy evidence regarding the possible advantages and hazards of the practice, these trials should include a variety of populations and account for confounding variables.

3. Standardization of methods: Develop standardized protocols and methods for vaginal seeding to ensure consistency and reproducibility across different healthcare settings. Standardization will help in comparing results across studies and improve the quality of research in this area.

4. Impact of antibiotics: Investigate the impact of maternal and neonatal antibiotic use on neonatal microbial colonization. Understanding how antibiotics affect the neonatal microbiome can inform strategies to minimize their impact on microbial diversity and balance.

5. Factors influencing microbial transfer: Explore other factors that may influence microbial transfer during vaginal delivery, such as gestational age, mode of onset of labor, and maternal health conditions. Identifying these factors can help in understanding the complexity of neonatal microbial colonization.

6. Microbial analysis techniques: Continue to improve and refine microbial analysis techniques, including advanced sequencing methods and bioinformatic tools. This will enhance our ability to accurately characterize the neonatal microbiome and identify specific microbial patterns associated with delivery mode.

2.7.2 Recommendations for clinical practice

1. Individualized Care: Provide individualized care to neonates based on their specific microbial colonization profile and other clinical factors. Recognize that each infant's microbiome is unique and may require tailored interventions.

2. Promote vaginal delivery: Encourage and promote vaginal delivery when it is safe and appropriate for both the mother and baby. Vaginal delivery exposes the infant to beneficial maternal vaginal microbes, which may positively impact their health.

3. Caution with vaginal seeding: Until more research establishes its safety and efficacy, practitioners should exercise caution when considering vaginal seeding. The potential risks associated with the practice should be weighed against the limited evidence of benefits.

4. Emphasize breastfeeding: As breastfeeding significantly influences the development of the infant's gut flora and general health, promote and support it. Breast milk provides advantageous substances that feed and promote the development of good gut bacteria.

5. Hygiene and infection control: Ensure strict adherence to hygiene and infection control practices during childbirth and neonatal care to minimize the risk of neonatal infections, especially for infants born *via* cesarean section.

6. Educate Parents: Provide expectant parents with balanced and evidence-based information about the potential impact of delivery mode on neonatal microbial colonization. Informed discussions with healthcare providers can help parents make informed decisions about their birth plan.

7. Interdisciplinary collaboration: Foster collaboration between obstetricians, neonatologists, microbiologists, and researchers to advance knowledge in this field. An interdisciplinary approach can lead to more comprehensive and clinically relevant research and recommendations. In summary, future research should focus on filling the gaps in knowledge regarding neonatal microbial colonization and delivery mode. In clinical practice, individualized care, promotion of vaginal delivery, caution with vaginal seeding, emphasis on breastfeeding, and adherence to infection control practices are key recommendations to optimize neonatal health. Collaborative efforts will continue to enhance our understanding of the intricate relationship between the neonatal microbiome and health outcomes [50–55].

This chapter reviews the existing literature on vaginal seeding, a practice aimed at replicating the microbial exposure of a vaginal birth for infants born *via* cesarean section (C-section). The review focuses on the impact of vaginal seeding on the neonatal microbiome composition, immune development, and health outcomes. Several studies have explored these aspects, providing insights into the potential benefits and controversies surrounding vaginal seeding. Studies have reported varying results concerning the impact of vaginal seeding on the neonatal microbiome. Some suggest that vaginal seeding can lead to an increased abundance of beneficial bacteria, similar to those found in infants born vaginally. However, methodological differences among studies may contribute to inconsistencies in findings. More well-controlled studies with standardized protocols are needed to further clarify the effects of vaginal seeding on the neonatal microbiome.

Vaginal seeding has been investigated for its potential role in promoting immune maturation in newborns. Some studies indicate that it may influence immune cell populations and cytokine profiles, contributing to immune tolerance. Nevertheless, the clinical significance and long-term implications of these immune changes remain unclear and require further investigation.

Observational studies have suggested associations between vaginal seeding and reduced risks of certain health conditions such as allergies, asthma, and autoimmune disorders. However, evidence in this area is limited and based on small-scale studies or anecdotal reports. Large-scale and well-designed studies, including randomized controlled trials, are necessary to evaluate the potential benefits and long-term effects of vaginal seeding on health outcomes [56–63].

The review identifies several gaps in the current knowledge about vaginal seeding. These include the lack of standardized protocols, variations in vaginal seeding practices, small sample sizes, limited long-term follow-up studies, and insufficient diversity among study populations. Safety concerns, mechanistic understanding, and the need for broader well-controlled research are also highlighted as areas that require attention..

In conclusion, while the existing literature provides some evidence suggesting the potential benefits of vaginal seeding, it also underscores the need for further research. Standardized protocols, larger sample sizes, diverse study populations, and extended follow-up periods are essential to establish a clearer understanding of vaginal seeding's impact on the neonatal microbiome, immune development, and health outcomes. Addressing these gaps will help healthcare professionals make more informed decisions about the use of vaginal seeding and its potential role in promoting neonatal health and well-being.

2.8 Recapitulation of the importance and implications of the research

The research on vaginal seeding holds significant importance in the field of neonatal health and microbial development. Recapitulating the key findings and implications of the research sheds light on the potential impact and controversies surrounding this practice [56–63].

The neonatal microbiome plays a crucial role in immune development, metabolic processes, and overall health outcomes. Understanding how vaginal seeding influences the neonatal microbiome composition can have far-reaching implications for neonatal health and disease prevention. With an increasing number of births occurring *via* cesarean section, exploring interventions such as vaginal seeding becomes crucial to promote microbial diversity and mimic the benefits of vaginal delivery. This research addresses the potential differences in the microbiome between infants, born *via* C-section and those delivered vaginally. Investigating the impact of vaginal seeding on immune development provides insights into potential strategies to promote immune tolerance and reduce the risk of immune-related disorders in later life. Exploring associations between vaginal seeding and reduced risks of allergies, asthma, and autoimmune disorders highlights the potential long-term health benefits of this practice. However, due to limited evidence, further research is necessary to draw definitive conclusions [56–63].

The findings of this research may influence clinical practice by encouraging healthcare professionals to consider vaginal seeding as an option for infants born *via* C-section. However, due to safety concerns and the need for more robust evidence, further research and standardized protocols are necessary before widespread adoption. The research underscores the importance of educating pregnant women about the potential benefits and risks of vaginal seeding. Clear communication with expectant mothers can help them make informed decisions about their birth plan and understand the implications of various delivery methods.

Identifying gaps in the current knowledge highlights the need for future research priorities. Larger-scale studies with diverse populations, long-term follow-up, and standardized protocols will contribute to a more comprehensive understanding of vaginal seeding's effects [56–63].

2.9 Final remarks and closing thoughts

In conclusion, the research on vaginal seeding represents a compelling area of investigation with potential implications for neonatal health and development. The neonatal microbiome and immune system are critical factors in shaping an infant's health and well-being and understanding how vaginal seeding influences these aspects is of utmost importance.

The conclusions drawn from the body of material already in existence indicate the potential advantages of vaginal seeding in promoting a microbiome composition that is similar to that of vaginally delivered children. Such a procedure may promote immunological development and maybe lower the risk of developing certain diseases in later life. However, it is essential to recognize that the evidence is currently limited and often inconsistent, necessitating further research with standardized protocols and larger sample sizes to validate these findings [56–63].

The research also emphasizes the importance of addressing gaps in our current knowledge. Long-term follow-up studies, inclusion of diverse populations, and standardized procedures are necessary to draw definitive conclusions about the safety and effectiveness of vaginal seeding. Moreover, ethical considerations surrounding informed consent, safety protocols, and potential risks should remain at the forefront of any research or clinical implementation [56–63].

The idea of vaginal seeding has potential, but caution must be used to prevent oversimplifying results until more conclusive data are available. The medical community should collaborate to prioritize research efforts in this field to ensure that decisions concerning vaginal seeding are evidence-based and prioritize the well-being of newborns and their mothers [55–63]. In closing, the exploration of vaginal seeding represents a fascinating avenue of research that has the potential to impact the future of neonatal care positively. By advancing our understanding of the neonatal microbiome and immune development, we can pave the way for more personalized and effective interventions. Continued investigation, collaboration, and critical evaluation will be crucial in unlocking the full potential of vaginal seeding and its implications for neonatal health and long-term outcomes. Ultimately, with evidence-based knowledge, we can strive to provide the best possible start in life for every newborn and support their journey toward a healthy and thriving future.

Author details

Panagiotis Tsikouras*, Xanthi Anthoulaki, Efthimios Oikonomou, Anastasia Bothou, Konstantinos Nikolettos, Alexios Alexiou, Dimitrios Kyriakou, Theopi Nalbanti, Sonia Kotanidou, Nektaria Kritsotaki, Natalia Sahnova, Aise Chatzi Ismail, Vlasios Spanakis, Georgios Iatrakis and Nikolaos Nikolettos
Department of Obstetrics and Gynecology, Democritus University of Thrace, Greece

*Address all correspondence to: tsikouraspanagiotis@gmail.com

References

[1] Dunlop AL, Mulle JG, Ferranti EP, Edwards S, Dunn AB, Corwin EJ. Maternal microbiome and pregnancy outcomes that impact infant health: A review. Advances in Neonatal Care. 2015;**15**:377-385

[2] Hu J, Nomura Y, Bashir A, Fernandez-Hernandez H, Itzkowitz S, Pei Z, et al. Diversified microbiota of meconium is affected by maternal diabetes status. PLoS One. 2013;**8**:e78257

[3] Aagaard K, Ma J, Antony KM, Ganu R, Petrosino J, Versalovic J. The placenta harbors a unique microbiome. Science Translational Medicine. 2014;**6**:237ra65

[4] Genc M, Onderdonk A. Endogenous bacterial flora in pregnant women and the influence of maternal genetic variation. BJOG: An International Journal of Obstetrics and Gynaecology. 2011;**118**:154-163

[5] Marchesi JR, Ravel J. The vocabulary of microbiome research: A proposal. Microbiome. 2015;**3**:31. DOI: 10.1186/s40168-015-0094-5

[6] Miller E, Beasley D, Dunn R, Archie E. Lactobacilli dominance and vaginal pH: Why is the human vaginal microbiome unique? Frontiers in Microbiology. 2016;**7**:1936. DOI: 10.3389/fmicb.2016.01936

[7] Mølgard-Nielsen D, Svanström H, Melbye M, Hviid A, Pasternak B. Association between use of oral fluconazole during pregnancy and risk of spontaneous abortion and stillbirth. Journal of the American Medical Association. 2016;**315**:58-67

[8] Aldunate M, Srbinovski D, Hearps AC, Latham CF, Ramsland PA, Gugasyan R, et al. Antimicrobial and immune modulatory effects of lactic acid and short chain fatty acids produced by vaginal microbiota associated with eubiosis and bacterial vaginosis. Frontiers in Physiology. 2015;**6**:164. DOI: 10.3389/fphys.2015.00164

[9] Witkin SS. The vaginal microbiome, vaginal anti-microbial defence mechanisms and the clinical challenge of reducing infection-related preterm birth. BJOG: An International Journal of Obstetrics and Gynaecology. 2015;**122**:213-218. DOI: 10.1111/1471-0528.13115

[10] Nuriel-Ohayon M, Neuman HKO. Microbial changes during pregnancy, birth, and infancy. Frontiers in Microbiology. 2016;**7**:1031

[11] Stumpf RM, Wilson BA, Rivera A, Yildirim S, Yeoman CJ, Polk JD, et al. The primate vaginal microbiome: Comparative context and implications for human health and disease. American Journal of Physical Anthropology. 2013;**152**:119-134. DOI: 10.1002/ajpa.22395

[12] Ravel J, Gajer P, Abdo Z, Karlebach S, Gorle R, Russell J, et al. Vaginal microbiome of reproductive-age women. Proceedings of the National Academy of Sciences of the United States of America. 2011;**108**:4680-4687

[13] MacIntyre DA, Chandiramani M, Lee YS, Kindinger L, Smith A, Angelopoulos N, et al. The vaginal microbiome during pregnancy and the postpartum period in a European population. Scientific Reports. 2015;**5**:8988. DOI: 10.1038/srep08988

[14] Petrova MI, Reid G, Vaneechoutte M, Lebeer S. Lactobacillus iners: Friend or foe? Trends in Microbiology.

2017;**25**:182-191. DOI: 10.1016/j.tim.2016.11.007

[15] Lee SK, Kim CJ, Kim DJ, Kang JH. Immune cells in the female reproductive tract. Immune Network. 2015;**15**:16-26. DOI: 10.4110/in.2015.15.1.16

[16] Keelan JA. Pharmacological inhibition of inflammatory pathways for the prevention of preterm birth. Journal of Reproductive Immunology. 2011;**88**:176-184

[17] Araos R, D'Agata EMC. The human microbiota and infection prevention. Infection Control & Hospital Epidemiology. May 2019;**40**(5):585-589. DOI: 10.1017/ice.2019.28. Epub 2019 Feb 19. PMID: 30777586

[18] ACOG Committee Opinion. Vaginal seeding. The American College of Obstetricians and Gynecologists. 2017;**130**(5):e274-e278

[19] Van De Wijgert JHHM, Borgdor H, Verhelst R, Crucitti T, Francis S, Verstraelen H, et al. The vaginal microbiota: What have we learned after a decade of molecular characterization? PLoS One. 2014;**9**:e105998

[20] Chen C, Song X, Wei W, Zhong H, Dai J, Lan Z, et al. The microbiota continuum along the female reproductive tract and its relation to uterine-related diseases. Nature Communications. 2017;**8**:875

[21] Ran G, Mladenovi V. Microbiological aspects of vulvovaginitis in prepubertal girls. European Journal of Pediatrics. 2012;**171**:1203-1208

[22] Yamamoto T, Zhou X, Williams CJ, Hochwalt A, Forney LJ. Bacterial populations in the vaginas of healthy adolescent women. Journal of Pediatric and Adolescent Gynecology. 2009;**22**:11-18

[23] Al-Baghdadi O, Ewies AAA. Topical estrogen therapy in the management of postmenopausal vaginal atrophy: An up-to-date overview. Climacteric. 2009;**12**(91):105

[24] Braundmeier AG, Lenz KM, Inman KS, Chia N, Jeraldo P, Walther António MRS, et al. Individualized medicine and the microbiome in reproductive tract. Frontiers in Physiology. 2015;**6**:97

[25] Mills BB. Vaginitis: Beyond the basics. Clinical Obstetrics and Gynecology. 2017;**44**:159-177

[26] Rice A, ElWerdany M, Hadoura E, Mahmood T. Vaginal discharge. Obstetrics, Gynaecology and Reproductive Medicine. 2016;**26**:317-323

[27] Donders GG, Bellen G, Grinceviciene S, Ruban K, Vieira-Baptista P. Aerobic vaginitis: No longer a stranger. Research in Microbiology. Nov-Dec 2017;**168**(9-10): 845-858. DOI: 10.1016/j.resmic.2017.04.004. Epub 2017 May 11. PMID: 28502874

[28] Beigi RH, Yudin MH, Cosentino L, Meyn LA, Hillier SL. Cytokines, pregnancy, and bacterial vaginosis: Comparison of levels of cervical cytokines in pregnant and nonpregnant women with bacterial vaginosis. The Journal of Infectious Diseases. 2007;**196**:1355-1360

[29] Simhan HN, Krohn MA. First-trimester cervical inflammatory milieu and subsequent early preterm birth. Am J Obstet Gynecol. 2009; 200:377e1-4. Of vaginal microbial communities in adult healthy women using cultivation independent methods. Microbiology. 2004;**150**(Pt 8):2565-2573

[30] Gajer P, Brotman RM, Bai G, Sakamoto J, Ursel ME, Zhong X, et al.

Temporal dynamics of the human vaginal microbiota. Science Translational Medicine. 2012;**4**(132):132ra52. DOI: 10.1126/scitranslmed.3003605

[31] Witkin SS, Mendes-Soares H, Linhares IM, Jayaram A, Ledger WJ, Forney LJ. Influence of vaginal bacteria and D-and L-lactic acid isomers on vaginal extracellular matrix metalloproteinase inducer: Implications for protection against upper genital tract infections. MBio. 2013;**4**:e0046013. DOI: 10.1128/mBio.00460-13

[32] O'Hanlon DE, Lanier BR, Moench TR, Cone RA. Cervicovaginal fluid and semen block the microbicidal activity of hydrogen peroxide produced by vaginal lactobacilli. BMC Infectious Diseases. 2010;**10**:120. DOI: 10.1186/1471-2334-10-120

[33] O'Hanlon DE, Moench TR, Cone RA. In vaginal fluid, bacteria associated with bacterial vaginosis can be suppressed with lactic acid but not hydrogen peroxide. BMC Infectious Diseases. 2011;**11**:200. DOI: 10.1186/1471-2334-11-200

[34] Selle K, Klaenhammer TR. Genomic and phenotypic evidence for probiotic influences of lactobacillus Gasseri on human health. FEMS Microbiology Reviews. 2013;**37**(6):915-935. DOI: 10.1111/15746976.12021

[35] Mendes-Soares H, Suzuki H, Hickey RJ, Fornay LJ. Comparative functional genomics of lactobacillus spp. reveals possible mechanisms for specialization of vaginal lactobacilli to their environment. Journal of Bacteriology. Apr 2014;**196**(7):1458-1470. DOI: 10.1128/JB.01439-13. Epub 2014 Jan 31. PMID: 24488312

[36] O'Sullivan O, O'Callaghan J, Sangrador-Vegas A, McAuliffe O, Slattery L, Kaleta P, et al. Comparative genomics of lactic acid bacteria reveals a niche-specific gene set. BMC Microbiology. 2009;**9**:50. DOI: 10.1186/1471-2180-9-50

[37] Huang B, Fettweis JM, Brooks P, Jefferson KK, Buck GA. The changing landscape of the vaginal microbiome. Clinics in Laboratory Medicine. 2014;**34**:747-761

[38] Fettweis JM, Brooks JP, Serrano MG, Sheth NU, Girerd PH, Edwards DJ, et al. Differences in vaginal microbiome in African American women versus women of European ancestry. Microbiology. 2014;**160**:2272-2282. DOI: 10.1099/mic.0.081034-0

[39] Macklaim JM, Cohen CR, Donders G, Gloor GB, Hill JE, Parham GP, et al. Exploring a road map to counter misconceptions about the cervicovaginal microbiome and disease. Reproductive Sciences. 2012;**19**:1154-1162

[40] Dermendjiev T, Pehlivanov B, Hadjieva K, Stanev S. Epidemiological, clinical and microbiological findings in women with aerobic vaginitis. Akusherstvo i Ginekologiia. 2015;**54**:4-8

[41] Tansarli GS, Kostaras EK, Athanasiou S, Falagas ME. Prevalence and treatment of aerobic vaginitis among non-pregnant women: Evaluation of the evidence for an underestimated clinical entity. European Journal of Clinical Microbiology & Infectious Diseases. 2013;**32**:977-984

[42] Rumyantseva TA, Bellen G, Savochkina YA, Guschin AE, Donders GG. Diagnosis of aerobic vaginitis by quantitative real-time PCR. Archives of Gynecology and Obstetrics. 2016;**294**:109-114

[43] Fan A, Yue Y, Geng N, Zhang H, Wang Y, Xue F. Aerobic vaginitis and

mixed infections: Comparison of clinical and laboratory findings. Archives of Gynecology and Obstetrics. 2013;**287**:329-335

[44] Mendling W. Vaginal microbiota. Advances in Experimental Medicine and Biology. 2016;**902**:83-93

[45] Geng N, Wu W, Fan A, Han C, Wang C, Wang Y, et al. Analysis of the risk factors for aerobic vaginitis: A case-control study. Gynecologic and Obstetric Investigation. 2016;**81**:148-154

[46] Mason MJ, Winter AJ. How to diagnose and treat aerobic and desquamative inflammatory vaginitis. Sexually Transmitted Infections. 2017;**93**:8-10

[47] Ginocchio CC, Chapin K, Smith JS, et al. Prevalence of trichomonas vaginalis and coinfection with chlamydia trachomatis and Neisseria gonorrhoeae in the United States as determined by the Aptima trichomonas vaginalis nucleic acid amplification assay. Journal of Clinical Microbiology. 2012;**50**:2601-2608

[48] Crosby RA, Charnigo RA, Weathers C, et al. Condom effectiveness against non-viral sexually transmitted infections: A prospective study using electronic daily diaries. Sexually Transmitted Infections. 2012;**88**:484-489

[49] Hughes JP, Baeten JM, Lingappa JR, et al. Determinants of per coitalact HIV-1 infectivity among African HIV-1-serodiscordant couples. The Journal of Infectious Diseases. 2012;**205**:358-365

[50] Workowski KA, et al. Sexually transmitted infections treatment guidelines, 2015. MMWR Recommendations and Reports. 2015. PMID: 26042815

[51] Roth AM, Williams JA, Ly R, et al. Changing sexually transmitted infection screening protocol will result in improved case finding for trichomonas vaginalis among high-risk female populations. Sexually Transmitted Diseases. 2011;**38**:398-400

[52] Andrea SB, Chapin KC. Comparison of Aptima trichomonas vaginalis transcription-mediated amplification assay and BD affirm VPIII for detection of T. Vaginalis in symptomatic women: Performance parameters and epidemiological implications. Journal of Clinical Microbiology. 2011;**49**:866-869

[53] Mohamed OA, Cohen CR, Kungu D, et al. Urine proves a poor specimen for culture of trichomonas vaginalis in women. Sexually Transmitted Infections. 2001;**77**:78-79

[54] Kingston MA, Bansal D, Carlin EM. 'Shelf life' of trichomonas vaginalis. International Journal of STD & AIDS. 2003;**14**:28-29

[55] Stoner KA, Rabe LK, Meyn LA, et al. Survival of trichomonas vaginalis in wet preparation and on wet mount. Sexually Transmitted Infections. 2013;**89**:485-488

[56] Sherrard J, Wilson J, Donders G, Mendling W, Jensen JS. 2018 European (IUSTI/WHO) international union against sexually transmitted infections (IUSTI) World Health Organisation (WHO) guideline on the management of vaginal discharge. International Journal of STD & AIDS. 2018;**29**(13):1258-1272

[57] Haahr T, Jørgensen SMD, Axelsson PB, Clausen TD. Neonatal Seeding after Caesarean Delivery: Hope or Hype Microbiologist. 2018. pp. 22-25. Available from: www.sfam.org.uk

[58] Anahtar MN, Gootenberg DB, Mitchell CM, Kwon DS. Cervicovaginal

microbiota and reproductive health: The virtue of simplicity. Cell Host & Microbe. 2018;**23**:159168

[59] Integrative HMP. (iHMP) research network consortium. The integrative human microbiome project. Nature. 2019;**566**:641-648. DOI: 10.1038/s41586-019-1238-8

[60] Serrano MG, Parikh HI, Brooks JP, Edwards DJ, Arodz TJ, Edupuganti L, et al. Racioethnic diversity in the dynamics of the vaginal microbiome during pregnancy. Nature Medicine. Jun 2019;**25**(6):1001-1011. DOI: 10.1038/s41591-019-0465-8. Epub 2019 May 29. PMID: 31142850

[61] Kindinger LM, Bennett PR, Lee YS, Marchesi JR, Smith A, Cacciatore S, et al. The interaction between vaginal microbiota, cervical length, and vaginal progesterone treatment for preterm birth risk. Microbiome. 2017;**5**:6

[62] Zhou SS, Tao YH, Huang K, Zhu BB, Tao FB. Vitamin D and risk of preterm birth: Up-to-date meta-analysis of randomized controlled trials and observational studies. The Journal of Obstetrics and Gynaecology Research. 2017;**43**:247-256

[63] Stafford GP, Parker JL, Amabebe E, Kistler J, Reynolds S, Stern V, et al. Spontaneous preterm birth is associated with differential expression of vaginal metabolites by lactobacilli-dominated microflora. Frontiers in Physiology. 2017;**8**:615. DOI: 10.3389/fphys.2017.00615

Section 4

Pueperium

Chapter 6

Postpartum Posttraumatic Stress Disorder

Maja Milosavljevic, Dusica Lecic-Tosevski, Snezana Rakic and Tijana Vranes

Abstract

Childbirth is considered one of the most important parts of women's lives filled with happiness and fulfillment. However, some studies have shown that delivery can be associated with psychopathological issues, postpartum posttraumatic stress disorder (PTSD) being the most serious one. Psychological trauma during delivery can be related to specific traumatic events (obstetrical complications) or postpartum PTSD could develop after "clinically normal delivery." The objective of our study was to examine the prevalence and risk factors for postpartum PTSD. One month after delivery 2.4% of 126 primiparous women developed PTSD and another 9.5% had clinically significant levels of PTSD symptoms. Obstetrical interventions were the only significant risk factor for the development of PTSD. It is important to assess the parturients for this disorder, which can influence the functionality of mother, father, newborn, the whole family, and, finally, the whole society.

Keywords: postpartum PTSD, traumatic delivery, obstetrical complications, posttraumatic stress disorder, peripartum

1. Introduction

In most countries and cultures, the experience of giving birth is considered a positive experience in a woman's life cycle. It is presumed that bringing a new being to this world opens the door to happiness and joy for a woman, her partner, and the whole family. In most cases it is so; if we exclude the expected "baby blues" during the postpartum period, the time after giving birth is mostly filled with positive experiences, and the childbirth itself remains a beautiful memory.

However, there are well-known situations where childbirth can be experienced as an unwanted experience filled with pain, trauma, and unpleasant emotions. It is only during the last few decades that the experts began to deal with this topic and scientific research began, in search of answers to what exactly leads to the experience of traumatic childbirth, what are its manifestations and consequences.

At the Institute of Mental Health and Obstetrics and Gynecology Clinic "Narodni front," situated in Belgrade, Serbia—for the first time, during the past decade, a study was conducted on traumatic childbirth experience, risk factors for its occurrence, and clinical consequences for the mother.

From the information found in literature so far, it is known that the consequences of a traumatic childbirth experience can be many. In the postpartum period, a woman who has given birth can have only a couple of posttraumatic stress disorder (PTSD) symptoms, or she can develop a clinical form of this disorder. A traumatic experience can, consequently, lead to a damaged attachment with the baby, impaired relationship between partners, as well as general dysfunctionality of a woman. Another possible consequence is the occurrence of secondary tokophobia.

Due to all of the above, the scientific observation of postpartum PTSD can open the door to a timely and adequate preventive work, better training of health professionals to recognize and offer help to women who have given birth and had traumatic childbirth experience, who are silently suffering hidden within the circle of their loved ones.

2. History

One of the first written documents that link traumatic childbirth experience and consequential psychological disorders dates back to the nineteenth century when it was described that "disturbing and scary dreams" after childbirth usually preceded the onset of melancholic stupor [1]. It was not until a century later that more intense studying of this phenomenology began. In 1978, academic literature mentioned 10 women that, after long and painful experience of giving birth, had nightmares related to the labor [2]. Some 10 years later, other symptoms of traumatic disorder had been described, such as symptoms of intrusion, emotional numbness, and dissociation, that appeared in women who had given birth, after complicated labors with anamnesis of infertility and complicated pregnancy [3].

Along with the change of diagnostic criteria in 1994, in the DSM IV classification trauma started being characterized as a subjective experience, and childbirth as subjective traumatic experience has become a topic of research when it came to frequency and etiopathogenetic mechanisms [4]. Childbirth started being treated as death threat, current or threatening injury, or current or threatening sexual violence (Criterion A of the DSM IV classification). During childbirth, a woman can feel like there might be immediate danger to her life or to the baby, regardless of whether it is clinically justified. A woman's belief that she is in danger can lead to psychological consequences [5]. According to DSM V birth trauma can meet criterion A (one is, directly or indirectly, subjected to actual or threatening death, serious injury, and/or sexual violence), and the symptoms are grouped as intrusion, avoidance, irritability, and negative changes in mood and cognition [6].

Postpartum PTSD and its clinical presentation were described in 1995 [7], and just a year later, PTSD after childbirth had a normal course from a clinical perspective [8]. It was not until after the year 2000 that more intensive research on postpartum PTSD began, mostly in more developed countries, and later in the rest of the world.

3. Risk factors for the onset of postpartum stress disorder and its frequency

It is significant to determine the definition of a "healthy or normal" childbirth. Medical model suggests it is a childbirth with no death occurrences, one without any medical interventions but also one where the mother, her wishes, and attitudes are appreciated. Childbirth is an extreme physical and psychological experience in the life of a woman, one which they can perceive either as a mild stress or a traumatic experience, depending on many factors. It differs from other potentially traumatic experiences because it is an occurrence a woman voluntarily goes through, and is a predictable, in most cases positive experience.

A number of factors can be linked to the onset of postpartum PTSD. As with PTSD after any other traumatic experience, risk factors for its occurrence can be classified in several ways: pre-traumatic (vulnerability factors and pregnancy itself), those related to the immediate effect of trauma (childbirth), and post-traumatic factors. Risk factors can also be classified into three groups: biological, psychological, and social. The specifics of risk factors for postpartum PTSD refer to the physiological changes that occur during childbirth, the circumstances in which childbirth takes place (most often hospital conditions), but also the active role of partners and health workers in the child-birthing process.

Risk factors that exist in the period before the traumatic experience are lower socioeconomic status of a pregnant woman and lower level of education, treatment of infertility, unwanted pregnancy, and previous traumatic experiences related to childbirth, as well as a history of psychological disorders (e.g. depression and PTSD) [9, 10]. Certain personality traits (neuroticism) can also be a risk factor for the onset of postpartum PTSD, as well as increased sensitivity to anxiety [11]. A history of sexual abuse, primarily in childhood, as well as pregnancies resulting from sexual abuse, are also pre-traumatic risk factors.

Factors present at the time of childbirth are as follows: stillborn child, spontaneous miscarriage, premature labor, or perinatal loss. The ending of childbirth, experienced pain, and social support during childbirth are also peritraumatic risk factors [9]. Obstetrical complications, such as vacuum extraction of the child, instrumental birth, emergency cesarean section, etc., are significant factors that can lead to PTSD.

The most stressful way of delivery for a woman is an instrumental vaginal labor, after that, an emergency cesarean section and normal vaginal labor, and the least stressful of all is planned cesarean section [11, 12]. The length of delivery and loss of blood during the entire event can be risk factors for postpartum PTSD. The feeling of having control over the delivery is something that can prevent the onset of PTSD, whether it's external control (over what other people are doing, the involvement of the mother in decision-making and sufficient level of information) or internal control (control over one's body and behavior).

Postpartum risk factors are inadequate social support (healthcare, support from a partner or family), newborn's temporary stay in intensive care units, additional traumatization, etc.

It is a known fact that postpartum PTSD can occur both after complicated and non-complicated deliveries, and it can even occur in women that had a "normal" vaginal delivery (delivery at expected time, with a healthy newborn). The subjective experience of childbirth itself is of key importance for the occurrence of posttraumatic stress disorder. Even when, medically speaking, neither women nor babies are in immediate life threat, some women will experience childbirth as a traumatic experience and later develop symptoms of PTSD.

Our study, which included 150 primiparous women that had a vaginal delivery, showed that there was no difference between the group of mothers with PTSD symptoms and those without symptoms in terms of sociodemographic characteristics and general clinical characteristics. The most important finding was that the group of mothers with PTSD symptoms had significantly more frequent obstetric interventions (vacuum extraction, forceps extraction) and pelvic presentation during labor [13]. However, it is still not known which biological and psychological factors are the most significant for the development of postpartum PTSD. Parameters of sympathetic activity (pulse and blood pressure) and serum cortisol concentration are mentioned in the literature as possible biological factors. In our study, we found no significant difference between pregnant women without symptoms and those with symptoms of postpartum PTSD in terms of body weight, systolic or diastolic blood pressure, or heart rate measured immediately after delivery (trauma) [13].

According to currently available literature, the prevalence of postpartum PTSD is from 3.1 to 4.7% [14]. It is important to point out that individual symptoms of this disorder can be noticed in a significantly larger number of women in labor, from 1.5 to even 33.1%. In our study, the prevalence of PTSD associated with childbirth was 2.4%, while 11.9% of women who have recently given birth had some symptoms of this disorder 1 month after childbirth [13]. The varying frequency of disorders in literature is a consequence of methodological inconsistencies. When the assessment was performed closer to the time of delivery, the frequency of disorders was higher. In accordance with the well-known fact of spontaneous recovery after a person's exposure to a traumatic experience of any kind, it has been shown that the prevalence of postpartum PTSD decreases as time passes after childbirth and that the clinical picture is then milder in intensity [13, 15]. If all of the above is taken into account it can be expected that a very small number of women will develop symptoms of chronic postpartum PTSD after giving birth. It is also known that the partners of women giving birth can also develop symptoms of postpartum PTSD, and according to some estimates, the prevalence is 1.2% [16].

4. Clinical presentation and comorbidity of postpartum PTSD

Postpartum PTSD is manifested through clinical symptoms that do not differ significantly from PTSD symptoms that arise after exposure to any other traumatic experience—with symptoms of intrusion, avoidance, and overstimulation.

The specifics of clinical presentation are directly related to the birth trauma itself. Avoidance symptoms are manifested through avoiding and neglecting obligations related to baby care, avoiding breastfeeding and gynecological check-ups, as well as sexual relations with the aim of preventing possible new pregnancies. Women who have recently given birth often avoid any conversation topics related to childbirth. If the next pregnancy were to occur, they would choose cesarean section as the method of delivery [17, 18]. Breastfeeding can be a trigger and remind a woman of the trauma she has experienced, which is why she may avoid it, but on the other hand, the healing effect that the act of breastfeeding itself can have should not be neglected. Successful breastfeeding helps the mother who has given birth to feel like a "good mother" and thus overcome the symptoms of postpartum PTSD faster and easier.

The specificity of symptoms of overstimulation in postpartum PTSD may resemble symptoms of excessive fatigue and normal physiological changes after childbirth. Women who have given birth can develop traumatic amnesia with the inability to remember the childbirth itself, and even if they do remember it, they often do so while feeling pain, fear, or sadness. Also, negative emotions such as shame or guilt due to the situation they are in can occur [5]. The course of postpartum PTSD is characterized by a reduction of symptoms over time [13], while a chronic form of this disorder can rarely occur.

Just as it does not differ from PTSD after any other traumatic experience in terms of clinical presentation, postpartum PTSD does not differ significantly in terms of comorbidities. Most often, this disorder is associated with depressive disorder [19], anxiety disorders, and substance abuse [9, 15, 20]. Postpartum depression and PTSD have several symptoms in common, including sleep disturbances, difficulty concentrating (concentration difficulties), a sense of a shortened future, lack of interest in normal life activities, and a sense of alienation from other people.

5. Treatment of postpartum posttraumatic stress disorder

Given the insufficient knowledge of the effectiveness of postpartum PTSD therapy, most recommendations are based on proven therapeutic procedures for treating PTSD after any other traumatic experience.

Normalization of the condition is a general therapeutic procedure that involves psychoeducation of mother about the symptoms of PTSD, as well as the fact that the symptoms do not reflect a personal weakness or lower value of the woman. Education on how to reduce symptoms of guilt and self-blame, as well as doubts about one's own competence as a mother, are further steps in therapy. The education of other family members, as well as the mother herself, is also important [21]. Evidence-based psychological treatment of PTSD is the implementation of cognitive behavioral therapy (CBT) and Eye Movement Desensitization and Reprocessing (EMDR) [22, 23].

Due to significant stigmatization, women with PTSD symptoms who recently gave birth rarely seek professional help. If they do ask for help, it is difficult for them to plan a schedule because of the new baby which makes it impossible to adhere to psychotherapy setting. They usually avoid taking the prescribed psychopharmaceuticals out of fear that the therapy will harm their baby through breastfeeding. In the Republic of Serbia, the Ministry of Health issued official guidelines for the use of psychotropic drugs during breastfeeding (available on the Ministry's website) [24]. The most commonly prescribed medication in the treatment of postpartum PTSD is antidepressants from the group of selective serotonin reuptake inhibitors (SSRIs).

6. The consequences of postpartum PTSD

The development of postpartum PTSD can have numerous consequences for the mother herself, her relationship with her child, her partner, and her general functionality. The child and the act of breastfeeding can represent a "threat" and a reminder of a traumatic experience for a mother who has recently given birth, which is why a woman can avoid any obligations related to the care and nursing of the child, as well as breastfeeding. Mothers who have just given birth usually spend most of their time with the baby, who actually reminds them of the trauma they experienced, and gradually they begin to feel that they are in a vicious cycle of remembering the trauma they want to forget.

Attachment is a phenomenon defined by Bowlby during the 1970s of the last century, as a child's need to bond with a person who cares for him, by which a sense of security and protection is achieved [25]. The primary figure of attachment is the mother, and based on these early experiences later in life, the child will later form emotional relationships and partnerships. Research shows that in mothers with postpartum PTSD, there is a disturbance in the emotional connection with the baby, which can have consequences on the subsequent development of the child.

Partnerships change in a way that a woman with PTSD symptoms can be "cold and reserved", avoid sexual relations and distance herself from her partner. Often, women avoid subsequent pregnancies, and if they do happen, they more easily opt for intentional termination of pregnancy and cesarean delivery.

7. Prevention of postpartum PTSD

Prevention measures for postpartum PTSD can be implemented on all three levels. Primary prevention would keep the disorder from happening (by timely identification of risk factors). Secondary prevention includes early identification of the disorder and the outset of treatment, and tertiary prevention includes rehabilitation of mothers who have already developed this disorder. The initial and basic step in the implementation of preventive measures is the education of health workers about the possibility of PTSD, risk factors, and the clinical course of postpartum PTSD, while the health workers in contact with women in labor [26] are expected to take on a more proactive role.

Primary prevention includes adequate psychophysical preparation of a pregnant woman for childbirth, as well as providing her with necessary information about the course of childbirth, possible obstetric complications, and medical interventions, making that information available at all times. Screening and identification of vulnerability factors take place during the procedure of obtaining detailed anamnestic data about previous pregnancies and their outcomes, previous traumatic experiences, and possible psychological disorders. Targeted screening is carried out if there is information about traumatic stress after childbirth. In that case, further steps should be adapted according to the ongoing and individual circumstances of each mother [27]. If there are real risk factors that could indicate the possibility of postpartum PTSD, a possible solution would be to offer those pregnant women a cesarean section as a way to end the pregnancy, noting in the medical documentation, as a mandatory sidenote, information about the special needs of such women during childbirth, with the possibility of providing additional care and support. In addition, it is important to provide women at risk with adequate pain control during labor. Satisfactory social support is an important factor in the prevention of postpartum PTSD [9, 10, 28].

Secondary prevention includes timely identification of traumatic stress disorder symptoms, acute stress disorder symptoms, or PTSD and providing adequate, evidence-based treatment. It is important to avoid psychiatrization, and attribute of the usual symptoms of fatigue, e.g. irritability, sleep disturbances, to PTSD symptoms. A woman who has recently given birth should be encouraged to talk about her experiences during childbirth.

Tertiary level of prevention is possible if traumatized mothers were to be monitored for a longer period of time with the aim of establishing a diagnosis of chronic PTSD and the need for further treatment [9].

8. Conclusion

Postpartum PTSD has symptoms of intrusion, avoidance, and overstimulation. With regular screening, it would be possible to detect pregnant women with problems and risk factors more easily and offer them adequate, evidence-based treatment on time. It is also very important to respect the personality of the woman giving birth, her wishes, and her attitudes, in order to establish compliance and implement treatment in the best way possible.

The fact that a certain number of women will experience their childbirth as a traumatic experience, which will result in their general dysfunctionality, disruption of their relationships with the baby and their partner, indicates that it is important to pay scientific attention to this phenomenon. It is necessary to look at postpartum posttraumatic stress disorder as an important link in the postpartum period, to focus the attention of experts and the general public in that direction. It is necessary to educate health workers as well as the women giving birth and their family members about the possibility of stress-related disorders and possible risk factors that can lead to the onset of that mental disorder. It is also necessary to destigmatize women who suffer silently, hidden from the health system. Carrying out prevention measures would achieve a goal of both mother and baby being well and taken care of.

Conflict of interest

The authors declare no conflict of interest.

Author details

Maja Milosavljevic[1]*, Dusica Lecic-Tosevski[2], Snezana Rakic[3] and Tijana Vranes[4]

1 Institute of Mental Health, Belgrade, Serbia

2 Serbian Academy of Sciences and Arts, Belgrade, Serbia

3 ECPD—United Nations University for Peace and Development, Belgrade, Serbia

4 North Bristol NHS Trust, Bristol, UK

*Address all correspondence to: maja.milosavljevic21@gmail.com

References

[1] Savage GH. Observations of the insanity of pregnancy and childbirth. Guy's Hospital Reports. 1875;**20**:83-117

[2] Bydlowski M, Raoul-Duval A. Un avater psychique méconnu de la puerpéralité: la névrose traumatique post-obstétricale. Perspectives Psychiatriques. 1978;**4**:321-328

[3] Moleman N, van der Hart O, van der Kolk BA. The partus stress reaction: A neglected etiological factor in postpartum psychiatric disorders. The Journal of Nervous and Mental Disease. 1992;**180**(4):271-272

[4] American Psychiatric Association (APA). Diagnostic and Statistical Manual of Mental Disorders. 4th ed. Washington, DC: American Psychiatric Association; 1994

[5] Kendall-Tackett K. Intervention for mothers who have experienced childbirth-related trauma and posttraumatic stress disorder. Clinical Lactation. 2014;**5**(2):56-61

[6] American Psychiatric Association (APA). Diagnostic and Statistical Manual of Mental Disorders. 5th ed. Washington, DC: American Psychiatric Association; 2013

[7] Ballard C, Stanley A, Brockington IF. Post-traumatic stress disorder (PTSD) after childbirth. The British Journal of Psychiatry. 1995;**166**:525-528

[8] Goldbeck-Wood S. Post-traumatic stress disorder may follow childbirth. BMJ. 1996;**313**:774

[9] Ayers S. Delivery as a traumatic event: Prevalence, risk factors, and treatment for postnatal posttraumatic stress disorder. Clinical Obstetrics and Gynecology. 2004;**47**(3):552-567

[10] Andersen LB, Melvaer LB, Videbech P, Lamont RF, Joergensen JS. Risk factors for developing post-traumatic stress disorder following childbirth: A systematic review. Acta Obstetricia et Gynecologica Scandinavica. 2012;**91**(11):1261-1272

[11] Verreault N, Da Costa D, Marchand A, Ireland K, Banack H, Dritsa M, et al. PTSD following childbirth: A prospective study of incidence and risk factors in Canadian women. Journal of Psychosomatic Research. 2012;**73**(4):257-263

[12] Grisbrook MA, Dewey D, Cuthbert C, McDonald S, Ntanda H, Giesbrecht GF, et al. Associations among caesarean section birth, post-traumatic stress, and postpartum depression symptoms. International Journal of Environmental Research and Public Health. 2022;**19**(8):4900

[13] Milosavljevic M, Lecic Tosevski D, Soldatovic I, Vukovic O, Miljevic C, Peljto A, et al. Posttraumatic stress disorder after vaginal delivery at primiparous women. Scientific Reports. 2016;**6**:27554. DOI: 10.1038/srep27554

[14] Kranenburg L, Lambregtse-van den Berg M, Stramrood C. Traumatic childbirth experience and childbirth-related post-traumatic stress disorder (PTSD): A contemporary overview. International Journal of Environmental Research and Public Health. 2023;**20**(4):2775

[15] Alcorn K, O'Donovan A, Patrick J, Creedy D, Devilly G. A prospective longitudinal study of the prevalence of

post-traumatic stress disorder resulting from childbirth events. Psychological Medicine. 2010;**40**:1849-1859

[16] Heyne CS, Kazmierczak M, Souday R, Horesh D, Lambregtse-van den Berg M, Weigl T, et al. Prevalence and risk factors of birth-related posttraumatic stress among parents: A comparative systematic review and meta-analysis. Clinical Psychology Review. 2022;**94**:102157

[17] Lapp LK, Agbokou C, Peretti CS, Ferreri F. Management of post traumatic stress disorder after childbirth: A review. Journal of Psychosomatic Obstetrics and Gynaecology. 2010;**31**(3):113-122

[18] Shlomi Polachek I, Huller Harari L, Baum M, Strous RD. Postpartum anxiety in a cohort of women from the general population: Risk factors and association with depression during last week of pregnancy, postpartum depression and postpartum PTSD. The Israel Journal of Psychiatry and Related Sciences. 2014;**51**(2):128-134

[19] Ayers S, Bond R, Bertullies S, Wijma K. The aetiology of post-traumatic stress following childbirth: A meta-analysis and theoretical framework. Psychological Medicine. 2016;**46**(6):1121-1134

[20] Howard S, Witt C, Martin K, Bhatt A, Venable E, Buzhardt S, et al. Co-occurrence of depression, anxiety, and perinatal posttraumatic stress in postpartum persons. BMC Pregnancy and Childbirth. 2023;**231**:232

[21] Kendall-Tackett K. Childbirth-related posttraumatic stress disorder: Symptoms and impact on breastfeeding. Clinical Lactation. 2014;**5**(2):51-55

[22] WHO. WHO Releases Guidance on Mental Health Care after Trauma. Geneva, Switzerland: WHO; 2013

[23] Lewis C, Roberts NP, Andrew M, Starling E, Bisson JI. Psychological therapies for post-traumatic stress disorder in adults: Systematic review and meta-analysis. European Journal of Psychotraumatology. 2020;**11**(1):1729633

[24] Nacionalne smernice za primenu lekova u periodu dojenja. Available from: https://www.zdravlje.gov.rs/view_file.php?file_id=1991&cache=sr [Accessed: July 21, 2023]

[25] Bowlby J. Attachment and loss. In: Attachment. Vol. 1. NewYork: Basic Books; 1969

[26] Milosavljević M. Prevalenca posttraumatskog strensog poremećaja (PTSP) u postpartalnom periodu i njegova veza sa nivoom kortizola u krvi [thesis]. Fakultet medicinskih nauka. Kragujevac, Srbija: Univerzitet u Kragujevcu; 2016

[27] White A, Saxer K, Raja S, Hall SL. A trauma-informed approach to postpartum care. Clinical Obstetrics and Gynecology. 2022;**65**(3):550-562

[28] Handelzalts JE, Levy S, Ayers S, Krissi H, Peled Y. Two are better than one? The impact of lay birth companions on childbirth experiences and PTSD. Archives of Women's Mental Health. 2022;**25**(4):797-805

Chapter 7

Histological Properties of the Chorionic and Basal Plates and Maintenance of the Mechanical Environment in the Human Placenta

Yoko Kato

Abstract

The human placenta is covered with the chorionic and basal plates, which face the fetal and maternal sides, respectively. Each plate shows its own characteristics in tissue structure so that these plates would have quite different mechanical properties: The mechanical environment of the placenta would be dependent on its position, a fetal side or maternal side. In the meantime, considering that the blood circulations in the placenta, the fetal blood flows in the blood vessels, which pass through the umbilical cord, chorionic plate, and villous trees, and the maternal blood flows in the blood vessels in the basal plate and intervillous space. The chorionic and basal plates would be necessary for the fetal and maternal blood circulations, respectively. In this chapter, the influence of the chorionic and basal plates on the mechanical environment of the placenta, and the fetal and maternal blood circulations, is explained.

Keywords: human placenta, blood circulation, umbilical cord, villous tree, Intervillous space

1. Introduction

The substances in the fetal and maternal blood, such as nutrition and gas, are successfully exchanged so that a fetus grows well. The fetal blood flows into the umbilical artery, circulates the blood vessels in the villous trees of the placenta, and returns to the fetus through the umbilical vein, while the maternal blood in the endometrial spiral artery flows into the intervillous space, corresponding to the space around the villous tree, and after circulating the space, returns to the endometrial vein. The fetal and maternal blood circulations do not share the space, but their substances are exchanged through the villous trees in the placenta. The condition of the fetal and maternal circulations would directly influence the substance exchange. Considering that the mechanical environment around these circulations could change the flow pattern, the environment would be modulated in order to keep the proper conditions of the circulations.

The umbilical cord shows the histological characteristics [1], which would be helpful to keep the mechanical environment suitable for the blood flow [2]. Also, the active contraction of the villous tree [3, 4], the contractile cells around the fetal blood vessels [5–8], expected to cause the contraction, have been reported. The computational models based on these previous reports [3–8] have been developed and indicated that the contractile system would be helpful for the fetal and maternal blood circulations [9, 10]. Moreover, it has been reported that the dilation of the spiral artery, caused by the loss of smooth muscle and elastic lamina, could modulate the maternal blood flow properly [11]. In the meantime, the deformation of the placenta and blood flow caused by the uterus contraction, evaluated by MRI images, has been reported [12, 13]. According to the previous report [14–16], the thickness and diameter of the placenta at the third trimester were about 40 mm and 200 mm, respectively. Comparing the placental size with the resolution of the MRI images (2.4 × 2.4 × 5 or 2.5× 2.5 × 6 [mm^3]) [12], these quantitative values would be helpful in the evaluation along the circumferential direction of the uterus.

The placenta at term is covered with the chorionic plate, marginal zone, and basal plate [17, 18]. The chorionic plate connects to the umbilical cord while the basal plate is next to the placental bed. The marginal zone is placed between these two plates. These regions, which are continuously connected with each other, show the two types of fibrinoid, the fibrin-type and matrix-type fibrinoid [17–20]. Also, smooth muscle was observed at the chorionic plate [5] and marginal zone [18]. The distribution was expanded to the basal plate [18]. The mechanical properties of the chorionic plate were evaluated by the elastic moduli and thickness in the amniotic and chorionic layers [21]: the amniotic layer, 1.90 MPa and 47 μm; the chorionic layer, 2.2 MPa and 185 μm; the entire layer, 4.7 MPa and 243 μm. The elastic moduli of the placenta were varied by the methods [22]: The elastic moduli at tension and shear were more than twice of those at compression. Considering that the amniotic and chorionic layers could influence the elastic moduli at tension and shear more than that at compression, the elastic modulus of the region surrounded by the layers would be much lower than those in the layers.

In this study, a computational model of the human placenta was developed in order to evaluate changes in the mechanical environment of the human placenta, caused by the elongation and contraction of the uterus. Based on the results, how the histological characteristics of the placenta assist the fetal and maternal blood circulations will be indicated.

2. Computational model of the human placenta and its analysis

The model development and computations were carried out by the finite element analysis software (COMSOL Multiphysics®, 6.1). The computational model of the human placenta, developed in this study, is shown by **Figure 1**. The morphological characteristics and mechanical properties of the components in this model are indicated by **Tables 1** and **2**, respectively. As **Figure 1** shows, the placenta is set as the ellipse (A), whose major and minor axes were based on the radius and thickness of the placenta at the gestational age (40 weeks), respectively [15]. The placenta was covered with the thin area (B_2) entirely, composed of the chorion (part of the chorionic plate), marginal zone, and basal plate. The thickness was corresponding to that of the chorion [21]: Because the thickness of the chorionic plate was larger than the sum of those at the amniotic and chorionic layers [21], the difference was evenly added to each layer's

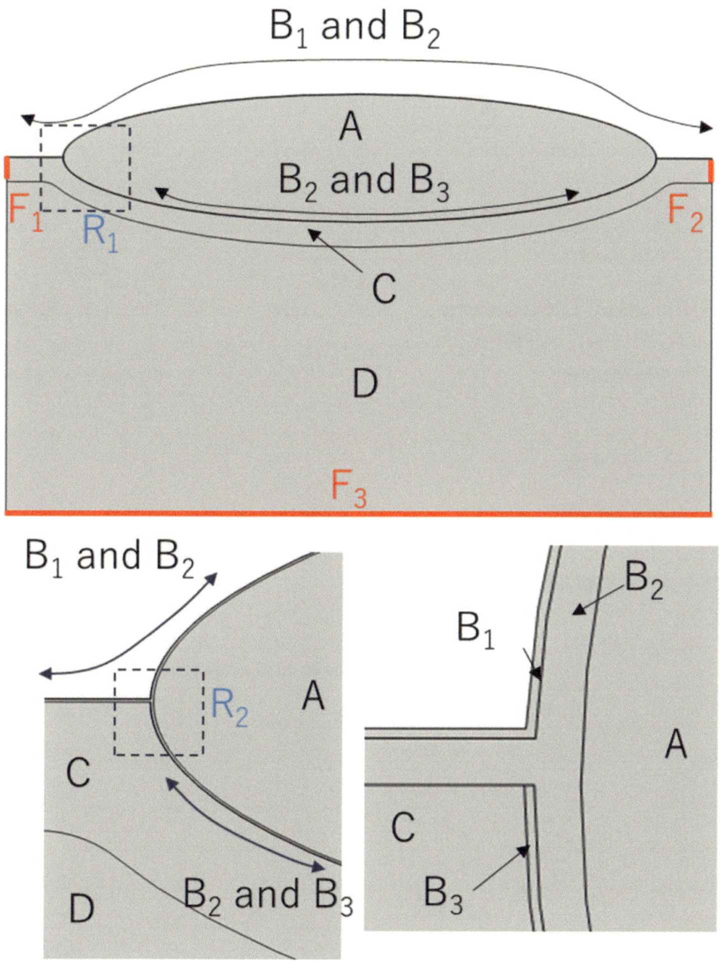

Figure 1.
A computational model for the human placenta and its surroundings, developed in this study. A, placenta; B1, amnion (chorionic plate); B2, chorion (chorionic plate), marginal zone, and basal plate; B3, boundary region between the placenta and myometrium; C, myometrium; D, surroundings. The details of the region R1 (broken lines, upper) and R2, part of R1 (broken lines, lower, left), are shown at the lower images (left and right), respectively. F1, F2, and F3 were fixed in all the cases.

thickness. Also, the region B_2 was surrounded by the two thin layers (B_1 and B_3): B_1, amnion (part of the chorionic plate); B_3, the boundary region between the placenta and myometrium. The thickness in B_1 and B_3 was the same as that in amnion [21]. B_1 and B_2, corresponding to the chorionic plate, were extended to the point, 24 mm from the ellipse A (about 10% of the major axis), keeping parallel with its major axis. Both ends of B_1 and B_2, F_1 and F_2 in **Figure 1** were fixed at all the computation. The region C, the myometrium, was put the thin regions (B_2 and B_3) with the thickness before labor [23]. Every region in the region C, including the side of the region A, and the region under the region A, was connected smoothly, with the radius of curvature, the same as its thickness. Considering that the uterus is constrained in the various ways, including cardinal ligament, broad ligament of the uterus ligament of ovary, and round ligament of uterus [26, 27], the region D (surroundings) under the region C (myometrium)

Region	Component	Type	Size
A	Placenta	Ellipse	Major axis = 104 mm [15]
			Minor axis = 22.5 mm [15]
B_1	Amnion (chorionic plate)	Layer	Thickness = 52.5 μm [21]
			Side = 24 mm
B_2	Chorion (chorionic plate), Marginal zone, Basal plate	Layer	Thickness = 190.5 μm [21]
			Side = 24 mm
B_3	Boundary region between the placenta and myometrium	Layer	Thickness = 52.5 μm
C	Myometrium	Layer	Thickness = 8.48 mm [23]
			Side = 24 mm
D	Surroundings	Layer	Thickness = 92.8–115.5 mm
			Side = 24 mm

Table 1.
Morphological characteristics in the computational model.

Region	Mechanical properties	
	Elastic modulus (Pa)	Poisson's ratio
A	5.0×10^4 [22]	0.3 [24]
B_1	1.9×10^7 [21]	0.3 [24]
B_2	2.2×10^6 [21]	0.3 [24]
B_3	1.9×10^7	0.3 [24]
C	1×10^7 [25]	0.499
D	1	0.3 [24]

Table 2.
Mechanical properties in the computational model.

was set. The bottom of the region D, F_3 in **Figure 1**, was fixed at all the computation. Assuming that the uterus could move to some degree, the elastic modulus of the region D was set much lower than that of the others. The elastic modulus of the placenta was corresponding to that at compression [22] in order to weaken the influence of the chorionic plate. The elastic modulus at chorion [21] was used for B_2. Because the region B_3 faces the maternal side, which is composed of the loose fibers and a complex vascular plexus [17], its elastic modulus was set at the same as B_1. While Poisson's ratio at myometrium was 0.499 for incompressibility as muscular tissue, that in other parts was 0.3, corresponding to gel [24], because incompressibility was not clear. **Table 3** shows the elongation and contraction of the uterus (Mode 1, Mode 2, and Mode 3). **Figure 2** shows the model with the triangular elements (305,336 elements).

The mechanical environment was evaluated by von Mises stress, the first principal stress, displacement, and the first principal strain. The distribution in each parameter was visualized. Also, the fluctuation of each parameter was evaluated along the lines, depicted by **Figure 3**.

Category	Mode	Fixation	Direction	Force/m (N)
Mode 1	Contraction	F_1, F_2, and F_3	From F_1 to F_2	8.48 [28]
Mode 2	Contraction		From F_1 and F_2 to B_{3C}	
Mode 3	Elongation		From B_{3C} to F_1 and F_2	
B_{3C}, the center of B3.				

Table 3.
Elongation and contraction of the myometrium.

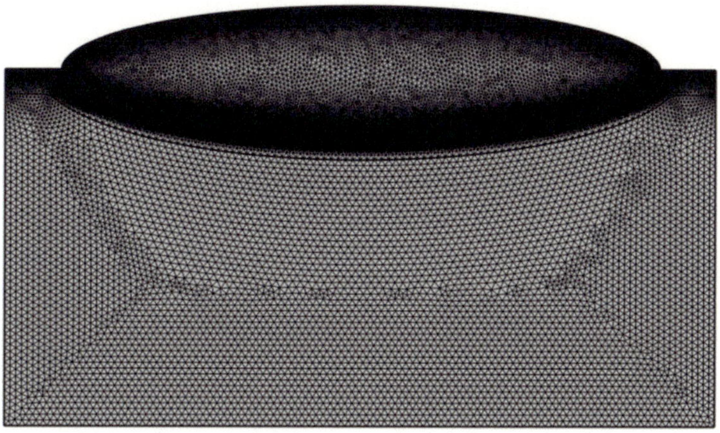

Figure 2.
Mesh in the computational model (305,336 elements).

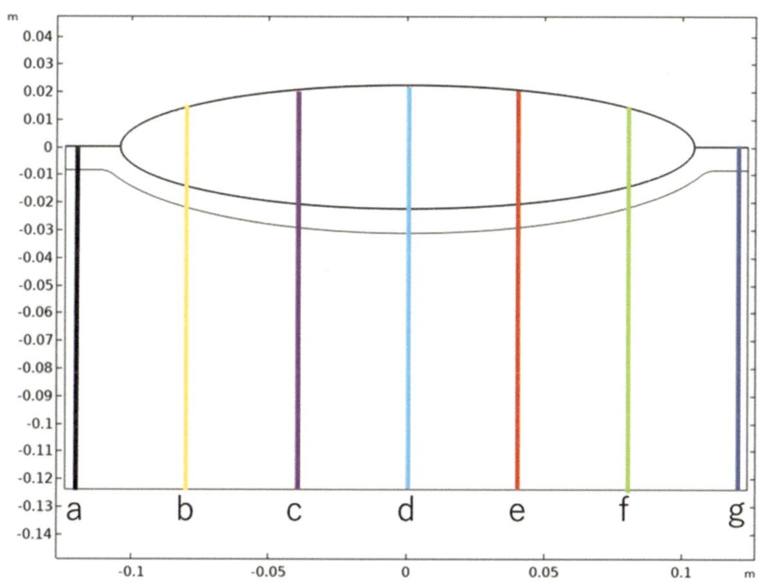

Figure 3.
Lines for evaluation in the mechanical environment of the placenta and surroundings. 7 lines (a–g), parallel with each other, were set 40 mm each along the horizontal direction.

3. Results

3.1 Von Mises stress and the first principal stress

Figure 4 shows the results of von Mises stress in each computation. While the shape of the placenta was largely deformed because of the myometrium contraction and elongation, von Mises stress in the placenta was kept much lower than that in the chorionic and basal plates, marginal region, and myometrium. Also, von Mises stress at these layers fluctuated largely. **Figure 5** shows the results of the first principal stress. As the results of von Mises stress, the first principal stress in the placenta

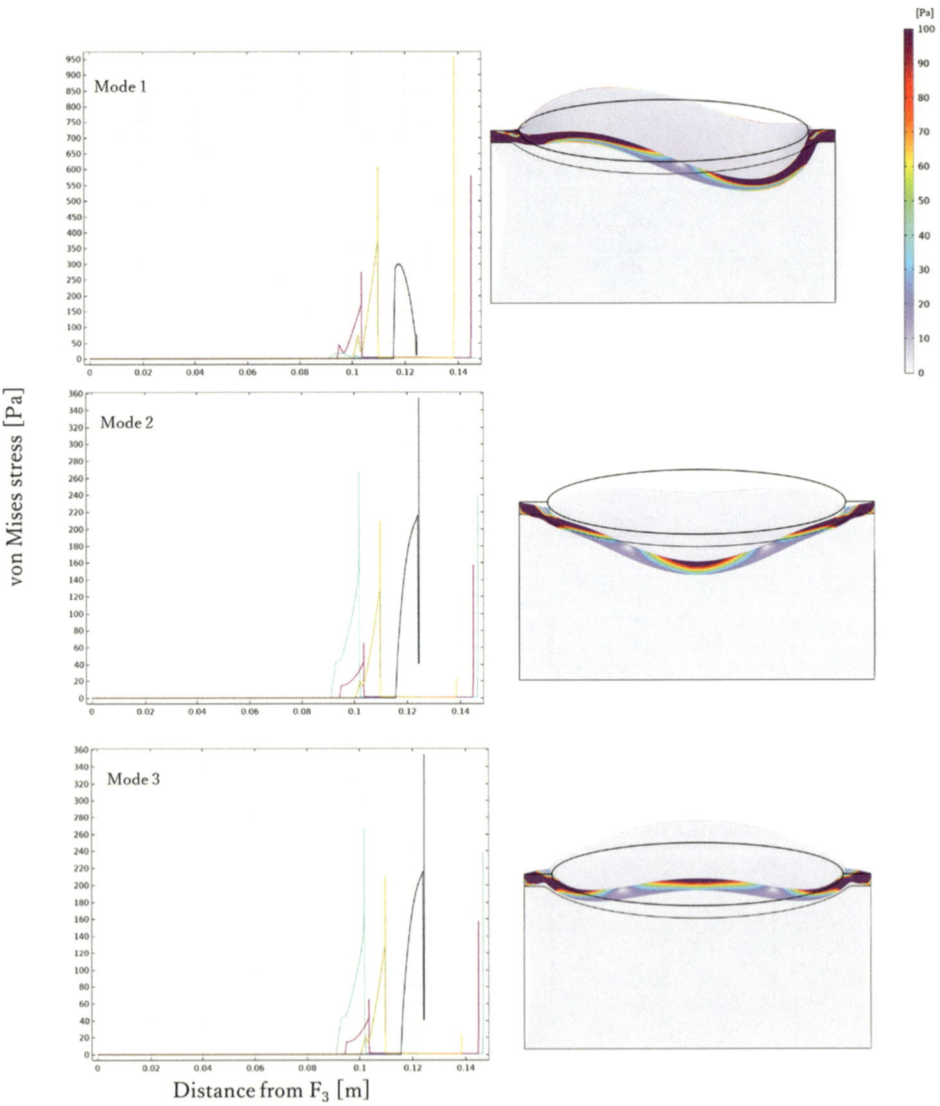

Figure 4.
*von Mises stress in the computational model of the human placenta and surroundings, caused by the myometrium elongation and contraction (Mode 1, Mode 2, and Mode 3 (***Table 3***)). The stress distribution is shown by the entire image (right), and the values along each line, indicated by* **Figure 3** *(left).*

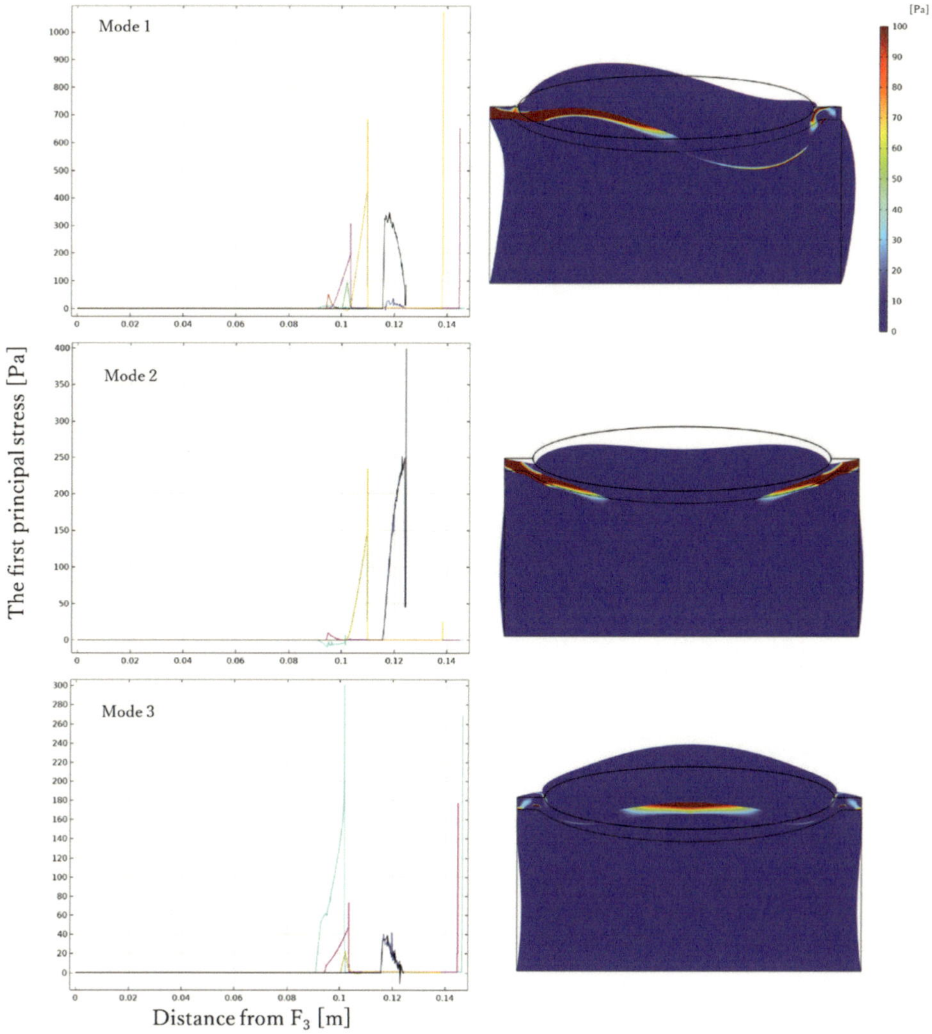

Figure 5.
*The first principal stress in the computational model of the human placenta and surroundings, caused by the myometrium elongation and contraction (Mode 1, Mode 2, and Mode 3 (***Table 3***)). The distribution of the stress is shown by the entire image (right), and the values along each line, indicated by* **Figure 4** *(left).*

was kept lower. The chorionic and basal plates, and marginal region, whose elastic moduli were much higher than the placenta, would prevent changes in the mechanical environment of the placenta. The stable condition in von Mises stress and the first principal stress would promote the effective usage of the perivascular contractile cells in the villous tree and chorionic plate for the fetal and maternal blood circulations.

3.2 Displacement and the first principal strain

Figure 5 shows the result of displacement in each computation. The deformation in the placenta at Mode 1 was much larger than that in other cases. The elongation and contraction the myometrium would cause various deformation patterns in the placenta so that the fetal and maternal blood could be stirred. As **Figure 6** shows, the first principal strain showed the same tendency (**Figure 7**).

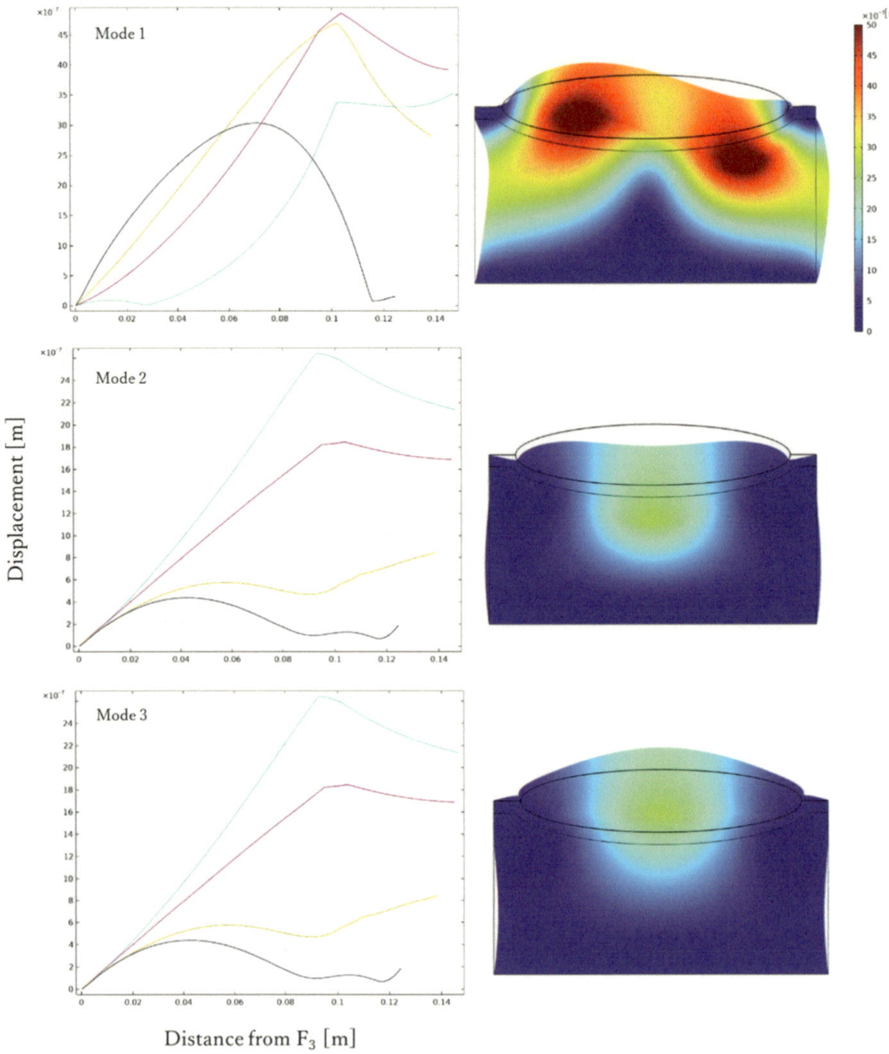

Figure 6.
*Displacement in the computational model of the human placenta and surroundings, caused by the myometrium elongation and contraction (Mode 1, Mode 2, and Mode 3 (**Table 3**)). The distribution of the displacement is shown by the entire image (right), and the values along each line, indicated by **Figure 3** (left).*

4. Discussion

In this study, the computational model of the human placenta and its surroundings has been developed, and the influence of the uterus contraction and elongation on the mechanical environment in the placenta was evaluated by the model. The mechanical load, such as force and stress, in the villous trees and intervillous space, which is corresponding to the placenta region in this model, would be stable although the large and various deformation could be caused by the uterus contraction. As the previous reports have indicated, the characteristic uterus contraction and elongation could deform the placenta [12, 13]. While the structural characteristics of the chorionic

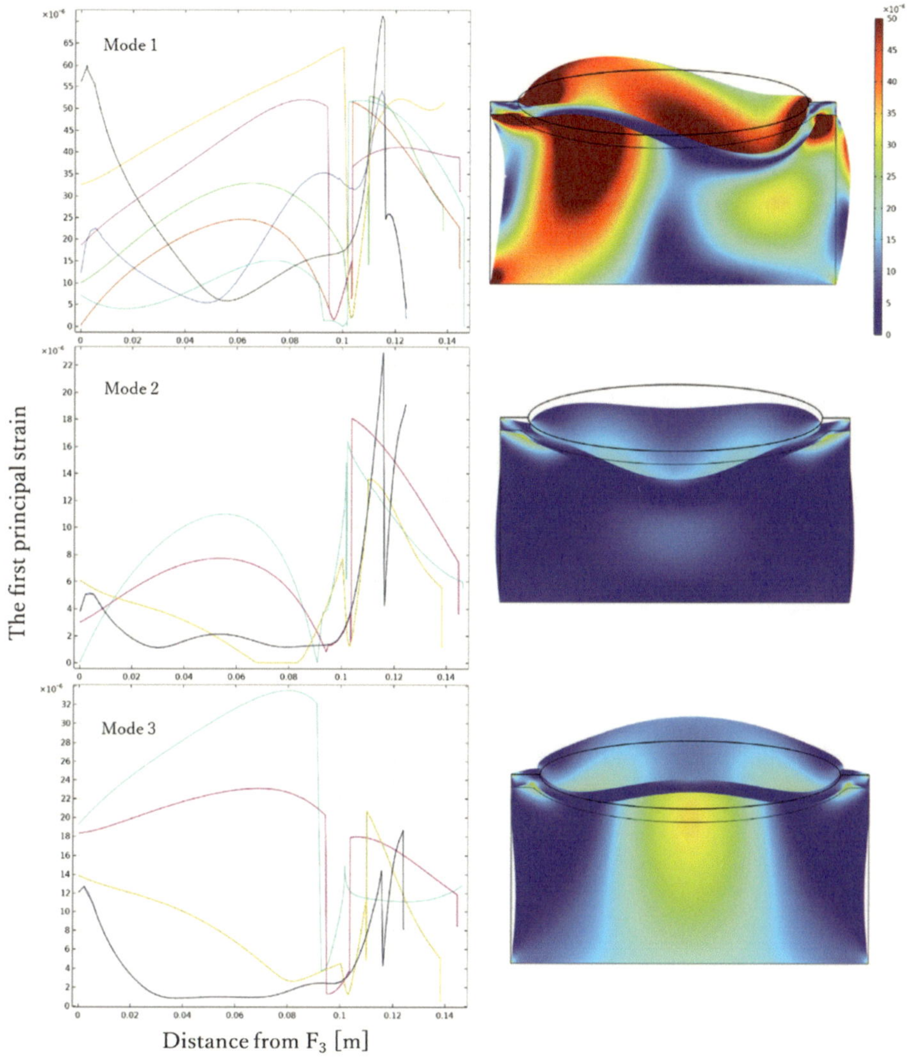

Figure 7.
*The first principal strain in the computational model of the human placenta and surroundings, caused by the myometrium elongation and contraction (Mode 1, Mode 2, and Mode 3 (***Table 3***)). The distribution of the strain is shown by the entire image (right), and the values along each line, indicated by* **Figure 4** *(left).*

and basal plates and its change along gestational age have been investigated [11], how these plates could influence the mechanical environment on the placenta has been barely examined. It has been reported that the smooth muscle in the marginal zone would actively influence on the uteroplacental vein [18], but its function for the blood circulation in the placenta has been barely examined.

While the thickness of the chorionic plate was just about 1% of the placental thickness [14–16, 21], the chorionic plate is composed of chorion and amnion, whose mechanical characteristics are quite different [11, 21]. Although the thickness and mechanical properties of the basal plate and marginal zone have been barely examined, these parameters in this model were the same as those of the chorionic plate in this model because they connect to the chorionic plate continuously. The results of this computational model have shown the importance of these thin plates for maintaining the mechanical environment of the intervillous space and villous tree.

The structural characteristics of the chorionic and basal plates and marginal zone has been simplified in this model. For example, amnion could be easily separated at "spongy layer" in the chorionic plate. This behavior would be mechanically important so that this layer will be taken into the computational model in the future. Also, fibrinoid, contained a lot in the placenta, including the chorionic and basal plates, is considered in the model development. Although the mechanical properties have been barely investigated, the estimation based on the previous reports [11, 19, 20] will be helpful.

5. Conclusion

The computational model of the human placenta and its surroundings, including the chorionic and basal plates and marginal zone, has been developed. The computation based on this model has indicated that the uterus contraction could cause the large deformation of the placenta, and mechanical load would be maintained so that the fetal and maternal blood circulation could be assisted by the contractile cells around the blood vessels.

Conflict of interest

The author declares no conflict of interest.

Author details

Yoko Kato
Faulty of Engineering, Tohoku Gakuin University, Sendai, Japan

*Address all correspondence to: ykato@mail.tohoku-gakuin.ac.jp

References

[1] Nanaev AK, Kohnen G, Milovanov AP, Domogatsky SP, Kaufmann P. Stromal differentiation and architecture of the human umbilical cord. Placenta. 1997;**18**(1):53-64. DOI: 10.1016/s0143-4004(97)90071-0

[2] Kato Y. Mechanical Environment in the Human Umbilical Cord and Its Contribution to the Fetal Circulation. London: IntechOpen; 2022. DOI: 10.5772/intechopen.106565

[3] Krantz KE, Parker JC. Contractile properties of the smooth muscle in the human placenta. Clinical Obstetrics and Gynecology. 1963;**6**(1):26-38

[4] Farley AE, Graham CH, Smith GN. Contractile properties of human placental anchoring villi. American Journal of Physiology. Regulatory, Integrative and Comparative Physiology. 2004;**287**(3):R680-R685. DOI: 10.1152/ajpregu.00222.2004

[5] Graf R, Langer JU, Schönfelder G, Oney T, Hartel-Schenk S, Reutter W, et al. The extravascular contractile system in the human placenta. Morphological and immunocytochemical investigations. Anatomy and Embryology. 1994;**190**(6):541-548. DOI: 10.1007/BF00190104

[6] Graf R, Schönfelder G, Mühlberger M, Gutsmann M. The perivascular contractile sheath of human placental stem villi: Its isolation and characterization. Placenta. 1995;**16**(1):57-66. DOI: 10.1016/0143-4004(95)90081-0

[7] Graf R, Neudeck H, Gossrau R, Vetter K. Elastic fibres are an essential component of human placental stem villous stroma and an integrated part of the perivascular contractile sheath. Cell and Tissue Research. 1996;**283**(1):133-141. DOI: 10.1007/s004410050521

[8] Graf R, Matejevic D, Schuppan D, Neudeck H, Shakibaei M, Vetter K. Molecular anatomy of the perivascular sheath in human placental stem villi: The contractile apparatus and its association to the extracellular matrix. Cell and Tissue Research. 1997;**290**(3):601-607. DOI: 10.1007/s004410050965

[9] Kato Y, Oyen ML, Burton GJ. Villous tree model with active contractions for estimating blood flow conditions in the human placenta. Open Biomedical Engineering Journal. 2017;**14**(11):36-48. DOI: 10.2174/1874120701711010036

[10] Kato Y. Influence of branching patterns and active contractions of the villous tree on fetal and maternal blood circulations in the human placenta. In: Aslanidis T, editor. Highlights on Hemodynamics. London: IntechOpen; 2018. pp. 27-43. DOI: 10.5772/intechopen.79343

[11] Burton GJ, Woods AW, Jauniaux E, Kingdom JCP. Rheological and physiological consequences of conversion of the maternal spiral arteries for uteroplacental blood flow during human pregnancy. Placenta. 2009;**30**(6):473-482. DOI: 10.1016/j.placenta.2009.02.009

[12] Dellschaft NS, Hutchinson G, Shah S, Jones NW, Bradley C, Leach L, et al. The haemodynamics of the human placenta in utero. PLoS Biology. 2020;**18**(5):e3000676. DOI: 10.1371/journal.pbio.3000676

[13] Hutter J, Kohli V, Dellschaft N, Uus A, Story L, Steinweg JK, et al. Dynamics of T2* and deformation in

the placenta and myometrium during pre-labour contractions. Scientific Reports. 2022;**12**(1):18542. DOI: 10.1038/s41598-022-22008-3

[14] Sun X, Shen J, Wang L. Insights into the role of placenta thickness as a predictive marker of perinatal outcome. The Journal of International Medical Research. 2021;**49**(2):300060521990969. DOI: 10.1177/0300060521990969

[15] Njeze NR, Ogbochukwu OJ, Chinawa JM. Correlation of ultrasound placental diameter & thickness with gestational age. Pakistan Journal of Medical Sciences. 2020;**36**(5):1058-1062. DOI: 10.12669/pjms.36.5.193

[16] Habib FA. Prediction of low birth weight infants from ultrasound measurement of placental diameter and placental thickness. Annals of Saudi Medicine. 2002;**22**(5-6):312-314. DOI: 10.5144/0256-4947.2002.312

[17] Burton GJ, Jauniaux E. The chorionic and basal plates. In: Baergen RN, Burton GJ, Kaplan CG, editors. Benirschke's Pathology of the Human Placenta. 7th ed. Cham: Springer; 2022. pp. 205-221. DOI: 10.1007/978-3-030-84725-8

[18] Nanaev AK, Kosanke G, Kemp B, Frank HG, Huppertz B, Kaufmann p. The human placenta is encircled by a ring of smooth muscle cells. Placenta. 2000;**21**(1):122-125. DOI: 10.1053/plac.1999.0455

[19] Kaufmann P, Huppertz B, Frank HG. The fibrinoids of the human placenta: Origin, composition and functional relevance. Annals of Anatomy. 1996;**178**(6):485-501. DOI: 10.1016/S0940-9602(96)80102-6

[20] Frank HG, Malekzadeh F, Kertschanska S, Crescimanno C, Castellucci M, Lang I, et al. Immunohistochemistry of two different types of placental fibrinoid. Acta Anatomica. 1994;**150**(1):55-68. DOI: 10.1159/000147602

[21] Oxlund H, Helmig R, Halaburt JT, Uldbjeg N. Biomechanical analysis of human chorioamniotic membranes. European Journal of Obstetrics, Gynecology, and Reproductive Biology. 1990;**34**(3):247-255. DOI: 10.1016/0028-2243(90)90078-f

[22] Weed BC, Borazjani A, Patnaik SS, Prabhu R, Horstemeyer MF, Ryan PL, et al. Stress state and strain rate dependence of the human placenta. Annals of Biomedical Engineering. 2012;**40**(10):2255-2265. DOI: 10.1007/s10439-012-0588-2

[23] Buhimschi CS, Buhimschi IA, Malinow AM, Weiner CP. Myometrial thickness during human labor and immediately post partum. American Journal of Obstetrics and Gynecology. 2003;**188**(2):553-559. DOI: 10.1067/mob.2003.77

[24] Greaves GN, Greer AL, Lakes RS, Rouxel T. Poisson's ratio and modern materials. Nature Materials. 2011;**10**(11):823-837. DOI: 10.1038/nmat3134

[25] Baah-Dwomoh A, McGuire J, Tan T, De Vita R. Mechanical properties of female reproductive organs and supporting connective tissues: A review of the current state of knowledge. Applied Mechanics Reviews. 2016;**68**(6):060801. DOI: 10.1115/1.4034442

[26] Ross MH, Powline W. Histology a Text and Atlas with Correlated Cell and Molecular Biology. 5th ed. Philadelphia: Lippincott Williams & Wilkins; 2006. p. 790

[27] Kaneko U, Kaneko K, Akita M. Nihon Jintai Kaibougaku (Anatomy in Japanese Human Body) (in Japanese). 19th ed. Tokyo: Nanzando; 2000. p. 420

[28] Arrowsmith S, Keov P, Muttenthaler M, Gruber CW. Contractility measurements of human uterine smooth muscle to aid drug development. Journal of Visualized Experiments. 2018;**131**:56639. DOI: 10.3791/56639